About the Author

Ron Lacey trained and practised as a social worker and psychotherapist. For 15 years he was an assistant director of MIND. Ron Lacey has written and broadcast on a wide range of mental health and related issues. In 1980 he co-authored a book on juvenile justice and in 1984 he co-authored the BBC book the *That's Life! Survey on Tranquillizers*. Amongst his other publications are the *MIND Special Reports on Psychiatric Drugs and Treatments*. His *Special Report on Tranquillizers* first published in 1983 was amongst the first publications to draw public attention to the problems of people addicted to tranquillizers, has been translated into eight languages and nearly a quarter of a million copies have been sent to people on request. For two years Ron Lacey was a radio agony uncle and his work has regularly been featured on television and radio programmes. He now works as a lecturer and freelance writer.

About MIND

MIND is the leading mental health charity in England and Wales. It works for a better life for people diagnosed, labelled or treated as mentally ill and campaigns for their right to lead an active and valued life in the community.

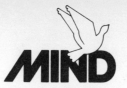

The Complete Guide to Psychiatric Drugs

A LAYMAN'S HANDBOOK

Ron Lacey

VERMILION
LONDON

Published in Great Britain by Vermilion
an imprint of Ebury Press
Random House
20 Vauxhall Bridge Road, London SW1V 2SA

Second impression 1993

British Library Cataloguing in Publication Data
Lacey, Ron
    The Mind complete guide to psychiatric drugs : a layman's guide.
    1. Psychotropic drugs
    I. Title
    615.788

    ISBN 0–7126–4778–3

Typeset in Trump Mediaeval by ⅀ Tek Art Ltd.,
Addiscombe, Croydon, Surrey

Printed and bound in Great Britain by
Mackays of Chatham PLC, Chatham, Kent

Contents

Acknowledgements

I owe a particular debt of gratitude to Derek Russell Davis, Emeritus Professor of Mental Health at Bristol University, not only for the generous help he gave me in writing this book, but also for the support and inspiration he has given to me and to my former colleagues at MIND over the years. Many people who have received help from MIND have benefitted from Derek's generous human spirit without ever being aware of it. I must also express my thanks to Professor Alec Jenner of Sheffield University for his generous help. It takes a particular generosity of spirit for eminent psychiatrists to help with a book which is so critical of psychiatry. If ever I or anyone I love needs the help of a psychiatrist I hope that someone like Derek or Alec will be there. My thanks also go to Rowena Webb at Ebury Press for cracking the whip when I got behind with my manuscript. During the twenty years in which I have been involved in mental health, I have learned a great deal about the strength of the human spirit from people who have suffered the pains of mental illness and its consequences in a community which often seems to be both mad and bad. I must thank my former colleagues at MIND, in particular, Tony Smythe, Larry Gostin, Tessa Jowell, William Bingley and Alan Salmon. I must also thank my wife Gillian for her support and forebearance. Emma Lacey and Rufus Lacey also deserve to see their names in print for all the love and joy they have given their parents over the years.

Ron Lacey.
March 1991.

Introduction

Each year MIND receives over ten thousand enquiries from members of the public on mental health and related issues. The majority of these enquiries are from people asking about the effects of psychiatric drugs, and most of these are concerned about their side effects. What has become increasingly evident from the enquiries is that people are not being given adequate information about these drugs by the doctors and psychiatrists who prescribe them. This guide fills an important gap; therefore, in describing the effects and side effects of all the psychotropic or psychoactive drugs which alter moods and behaviour. In addition, it puts this information into the context of what is known about prescribing practices, and in a language which everyone – not just medics – can understand. For this reason the drugs are referred to in this text as psychiatric drugs simply because this is the term that most laypeople use.

A quarter of all prescriptions dispensed by the National Health Service are for drugs which work on the central nervous system and affect mood and behaviour. The introduction of modern psychopharmaceuticals during the past 40 years has transformed and shaped our mental health services. Drugs are now central to the treatment of the variety of psychological states. The doctors and psychiatrists who prescribe these drugs are the senior and most influential professionals in our mental health services and the choices and decisions they make affect us profoundly when we feel so depressed or disturbed that we seek help outside the circle of our family and friends. The chances are that the sort of help they give us will be a prescription for one or more of the drugs listed in this guide.

The pharmaceutical industry in Britain is a major export earner and, as such, wields considerable influence. As Kenneth Clarke pointed out when he was Health Minister, a healthy pharmaceutical industry is important to the economic health of the nation. The drug companies spend vast sums each year to encourage doctors to prescribe their products – it has been estimated at £5000 per year of promotional material per doctor in the UK. In doing this they have an obvious responsibility to strike a reasonable balance between the desire to maximize profits with the welfare of the patients for whom their products are prescribed. Doctors receive a veritable barrage of information on drugs from the companies; inevitably emphasizing the virtues of the drugs, and international research has shown that the views of doctors on drugs are very effectively influenced by this. There seems, however, to be a professional reluctance on the part of doctors to give their patients anything more than the most rudimentary information about the drugs they prescribe for them. As far as any details of the side effects of the prescribed drugs are concerned, this reluctance is very worrying.

If you ask a doctor why he or she does not warn patients about a drug's side effects, that doctor is likely to advance one or a combination of the following reasons: 'I'm too busy and I don't have the time.' 'The patient lacks the knowledge to be able to put the information about side effects into its correct perspective.' 'If I tell the patient about side effects which they may or may not experience there is an increased likelihood that they will experience them, or imagine that they experience them.' 'Telling patients about side effects causes them unnecessary anxiety.' 'Patients seldom ask me about side effects.' 'My patients trust me enough to rely on my professional judgement.' Nearly all of these reasons for not warning patients about the possibility that they may experience undesirable side effects whilst taking a drug has some validity for some patients some of the time. However, many people *do* want this information and have a right to think that it should be made available to them. Under common law a doctor should obtain the informed consent of the patient for a given treatment. In reality that only means the doctor should give the patient a broad rather than a detailed understanding of the treatment. (For a fuller description of informed consent, see p. 186).

There is a worrying amount of evidence from both patients and published research studies that these powerful drugs are not always prescribed with the necessary care and sensitivity. In the literature of psychiatry a great deal of concern is expressed about the 'poor compliance' of psychiatric patients on treatment regimes, that is, patients who stop taking the medications prescribed for them. The prevailing view amongst prescribers seems to be that stopping medication is symptomatic of the mental illness for which the medication was first prescribed. This same literature also has many references to the problem of 'irrational prescribing' in psychiatric hospitals, drugs prescribed either in excessive doses or in 'cocktails' (a mixture of drugs) which make no clinical sense. Very little, if any, psychiatric research seems to have been done into the possibility that psychiatric patients' poor compliance to treatment might be related to the irrational prescribing practices of many psychiatrists.

The attitudes of many to psychiatric treatment are based on certain assumptions about those who receive it. It is commonly assumed that 'psychiatric patients' are by definition incapable of making rational decisions about their own needs. It is also assumed that the treatments offered for these badly defined 'illnesses' are universally effective and invariably benign. It is attitudes like these which make it extremely difficult for people diagnosed as mentally ill to play an active role in their own treatment and recovery or to have their concerns and complaints about treatment taken seriously. Such attitudes also serve the arguments of those who would like to extend the existing legal powers for the compulsory treatment of patients in mental hospitals to include patients in the community. In a minority of instances, these attitudes have some validity, but when they are applied as generalizations they constitute a grave threat to our well-being and civil liberties.

This guide is neither anti psychiatry nor anti psychiatric drugs. Psychiatrists and the treatments they offer are vitally necessary to the lives and well-being of many thousands of people. There are, of course, those who reject the whole concept of mental illness, and their contributions to the debate about the nature and causes of the variety of human conditions which are labelled as mental illness are important and interesting. But this debate has little relevance to the daily lives of most people currently receiving psychiatric treatment. There is also a small but vociferous minority who reject the concept of mental illness and see psychiatry as an agent of an oppressive state which seeks to enforce conformity regardless of its human costs. Their passionately held beliefs ultimately leave people who are tormented by strange and terrifying experiences without hope of relief. This guide is concerned with the practical day-to-day treatment of barely understood human distress by fallible professionals whose tools are imperfect drugs. The term mental illness is used in these pages because it is the term most people use to refer to those states of mind for which people seek and receive treatment from doctors, psychiatrists and other mental health professionals.

When properly prescribed the drugs used in psychiatry can relieve the misery of depression or terrifying hallucinations and delusions. They can help people lead lives which would otherwise be impoverished by profound despair or mental torment. But when prescribed without regard to their subjective effects or simply as a means of managing people by sedating them they can be a form of abuse. Like all other drugs used in medicine psychiatric drugs have effects beyond those for which they are prescribed. There is no such thing as a perfect medicine or 'magic bullet' which only attacks a narrow range of symptoms. The drugs used in psychiatry have a wide range of side effects which are often distressing, life-diminishing and sometimes even life-threatening.

Mental illness has distressing social consequences; to become a psychiatric patient often means losing one's credibility as a person. The language of psychiatry is unique in medicine in that it is also commonly used colloquially in order to abuse or discredit people. To be labelled as a 'neurotic', a 'depressive', a 'schizophrenic' or an 'hysteric' can mean being rendered invisible, and becoming subject to the often uninformed good intentions of others. Mental illness causes confusion, pain and distress to its sufferers and to those closest to them. The goodwill of families and other carers may be tested to the limits of its tolerance and beyond. When this happens, the real reasons both for using a drug and for the particular doses administered may be as much for the benefit of the carer as for the sufferer. While those around the sufferer may believe the drug is making him or her feel better, the sufferer may actually be made to feel a great deal worse by the effects of the drug. In these circumstances the mental patient is in a dangerously exposed position in which his or her protests are unlikely to be heard, and less likely to be acted upon.

Under the provisions of the 1983 Mental Health Act, patients subject to detention for treatment or assessment can lawfully be administered drugs by force. This can, and often does, involve patients being held down by nurses whilst drugs are injected into their buttocks. In some instances such forcible treatment may be necessary for the safety of the patient or of other people. However, the fact that powerful drugs may be administered forcefully to protesting patients imposes compelling moral obligations on those involved in such treatments. Perhaps the most compelling of all is the obligation to be sensitive to a patient's subjective experiences of a drug's effects. To be insensitive or indifferent to a patient's experiences is both negligent and callous.

Very few of those who prescribe and administer these drugs

have any direct personal experience of what it feels like to be on the receiving end of such treatment. The accounts of the few who have made interesting reading. A psychiatrist who suffered a serious depressive breakdown and was treated with anti-depressants described his surprise at the severity of the drug's unwanted effects in an article he wrote for his colleagues. In it he made this plea: 'It may be that the doctor can offer only symptomatic relief or none at all, but sympathetic enquiry itself can help the patient by legitimizing his complaints. It is easy for a depressed patient to become preoccupied with problems such as thirst, tremor and clumsiness, constipation or urinary retention, which may be bad enough to cloud the picture of an improving mental state. The staff should also bear in mind the effect that the treatment, as well as the illness, may have on cognitive function, as this may be an added distress for a patient who cannot appreciate what is happening or the fact the impairment is temporary.'[1] Significantly, the author wrote this article under the title of 'View from the bottom', which sheds light on the perspectives of the author as both psychiatrist and patient: as a psychiatrist he is at the top, as a patient, at the bottom.

The account of two psychiatrists who tested the effects of a commonly prescribed antipsychotic drug by injecting themselves with a very low dose (5 mg of haloperidol) also make fascinating reading.[2] They describe how they both experienced a marked slowing of thinking and movement, as well as profound feelings of inner restlessness. Each experienced a loss of will, a lack of physical and psychic energy. Neither felt able to 'read, telephone or perform household tasks of their own will, but could perform these tasks if demanded to do so. There was no sleepiness or sedation; on the contrary, both subjects complained of severe anxiety.' So affected by the drug were these researchers that both had to leave work for 36 hours. It is worth noting here that the dose they took was one-tenth of the initial dose recommended in the British National Formulary. It is also worth noting that antipsychotic drugs are often referred to as major *tranquillizers*.

In an article in an American magazine entitled 'I ate my mail', a general practitioner described how after becoming addicted to Valium he used to take the many samples of this

---

[1]Anon: 'View from the bottom', *Psychiatric Bulletin*, 14, p.452, 1990.

[2]Belmaker, R. H. and Wald, D.: 'Haloperidol in normals', *British Journal of Psychiatry*, 131, p.222, 1977.

and other similar drugs which he received through the post from drug companies. This article appeared 20 years ago, before doctors knew of or acknowledged the addictive potential of these drugs. Then withdrawal symptoms were conveniently dismissed as 'rebound anxiety', or as a recurrence of the symptoms for which the drug was first prescribed.

Prescribing in Psychiatric Hospitals – An Urgent Case for Treatment

There is a great deal of concern about the way in which drugs are prescribed by doctors and psychiatrists. The main areas of concern are 'polypharmacy', the prescribing of 'cocktails' of two or more similar drugs concurrently, and 'megadosing', the prescribing of drugs in extremely high doses. MIND receives thousands of complaints about the severity of side effects and the lack of attention paid to them by anyone involved in their treatment. When patients do raise the issue of side effects with their psychiatrists, quite often it is *they* who are seen to be the problem, rather than the side effects they are complaining about. There is evidence that points strongly to the possibility that over the years bad prescribing has substantially contributed to the problems which lead people to seek help from MIND.

A number of studies into the prescribing habits of psychiatrists in different parts of the country point to a very worrying state of affairs in which patients are needlessly exposed to the adverse and often dangerous effects of powerful drugs. One 1984 study of the prescribing of psychiatric drugs to in-patients and out-patients in a Birmingham psychiatric hospital revealed that just under half of all patients were receiving two or more drugs. Minor tranquillizers and sleeping pills were prescribed together with anti-depressant and antipsychotic drugs. A third of all patients receiving antipsychotics were receiving them both orally and by injection. A third of patients receiving antidepressants were not diagnosed as suffering from depression. The authors of this study expressed two principal areas of concern: the costs of such irrational prescribing to the health service and the potential dangers to the patient of bad prescribing. In the concluding paragraphs of their paper, they noted that the adverse effects of psychotropic drugs were becoming 'an increasingly important medico-legal issue'. It was, in effect, a warning to their colleagues that if they did not mend their ways of prescribing, they risked being sued by their patients.[3]

Yet another study of the prescribing habits of psychiatrists, published in 1987, reported that there had been no significant improvement in polypharmacy and overprescribing during the period 1983 to 1985.[4] A more recent study reported that between 1970 and 1983, polypharmacy and the use of multiple neuroleptics (antipsychotic drugs) had been reduced, the total dose of these drugs fell and the proportion administered by depot injection (that is, injections which are effective for a number of weeks) increased. Since 1983, however, some of these improvements had been reversed. Of particular worry in this study was the finding that the prescribing practices of a major teaching hospital concerned with psychopharmacological research had deteriorated. The authors noted that this poor standard of prescribing was 'unlikely to be a problem occurring on an isolated basis', and urged their colleagues not to use a 'production-line' approach to the prescribing of drugs. The numerous enquiries received by MIND's advice services strongly indicate that polypharmacy, megadosing and prescription production lines are far from rare in the experiences of those who receive psychiatric treatment as both in-patients and out-patients. If you are worried about the way in which your drugs are prescribed, you should raise this with your doctor, and if not satisfied, consider making a complaint (see p. 190).

Using This Guide

The purpose of this guide is to provide you with the information you need to play an active part in your own recovery. Much of the information in these pages points to the problems of psychiatric drugs and the ways in which they are prescribed. In using this information you must at all times remember that every decision as to whether or not to use a drug involves a judgement as to whether its benefits outweigh its disadvan-

[3]Edwards, S. and Kumar, V.: 'A Survey of Prescribing of Psychotropic Drugs in a Birmingham Psychiatric Hospital', *British Journal of Psychiatry*, pp.502–7, 1984.

[4]Clark, A. F. and Holden, N. L.: 'The Persistence of Prescribing Habits: A Survey and Follow-up of Prescribing to Chronic Hospital In-Patients', *British Journal of Psychiatry*, 154, pp.88–91, 1987.

[5]Johnson, D. A. W. and Wright, N. F.: 'Drug Prescribing for Schizophrenic Out-patients on Depot Injections. Repeat Surveys over 18 years', *British Journal of Psychiatry*, 156, pp.827–34, 1990.

tages. That decision is best made in collaboration with your doctor or psychiatrist. This guide is *not* intended to prescribe for you, its purpose is to inform the decisions you make with your doctor and with those closest to you who know you and the circumstances in which you live.

As will be clear from this guide, our mental health services have plenty of problems, many of which arise from the neglect suffered by them over the years. Mental health services have never had the prestige of other more glamorous, hi-tech areas of medical care, and people with mental illness have suffered from this neglect. In setting the information about psychiatric drugs within the context of the problems of the services which prescribe them, this guide seeks to promote a more informed discussion about the solutions to those problems. The principle of informed consent is not only important in the relationships we have with our doctors, it is equally important in our relationships with those who determine the priorities and policies of our health services. It is time that discussions about the needs of mentally ill people were based on the known realities and limitations of psychiatric treatment. Psychiatric drugs have a very important part to play in reducing the human misery caused by mental illness and distress, but only when they are used with proper care within the context of services which address our social, emotional and creative needs as complex, thinking human beings.

Introduction

Minor tranquillizers are prescribed to relieve anxiety and insomnia, as muscle relaxants and for the treatment of epileptic fits. They are also used by dentists to calm nervous patients. The most commonly prescribed minor tranquillizers are a group called the benzodiazepines, of which the two best known are Valium and Mogadon. Other less well-known and less widely prescribed minor tranquillizers which are not benzodiazepines are described on pp. 31–41.

Minor tranquillizers have been grossly over-prescribed and many thousands of people have become hooked on them. According to a MORI poll published in 1985 by the BBC, not less than 23 per cent of Britain's adult population has taken a minor tranquillizer at least once. Of those, 35 per cent, or 3.5 million people, had taken them for periods of four months or longer.[1] Four months is long enough to become hooked on them, and is also as long as tranquillizers are *known* to be effective. Some researchers estimate that approximately half of long term tranquillizer users will have difficulty in withdrawing from them; others put the numbers at one in eight, and others still at one in three. The MORI poll figure of 3.5 million long-term users suggests that between 435,000 and 1.75 million people may be hooked on minor tranquillizers.

The story behind the massive overuse of minor tranquillizers illustrates the dangers inherent in the attempt to provide medical solutions to the problems of living. Before drugs like Valium and Ativan became available, other frequently lethal 'minor tranquillizers' had already been overprescribed and overused. These were the justly infamous barbiturates which were discovered to be highly addictive and to have a potentially fatal withdrawal syndrome. They were also lethal if taken in

[1]Lacey, R. and Woodward, S.: *That's Life! Survey on Tranquillizers*, BBC Publications, London, 1985.

overdose, which could happen unintentionally. The discovery led to the setting up of a medical pressure group called CURB, which successfully campaigned for a dramatic reduction in the prescribing of barbiturate compounds, although to this day more people die of barbiturate overdose than of any other prescribed drug. The barbiturate scandal therefore created the ideal climate in which to launch a new 'safe' and 'non-addictive' minor tranquillizer which had 'few side effects'. That drug was chlordiazepoxide, better known by its trade name of Librium, the first of the benzodiazepine tranquillizers, and introduced in 1960.

Librium was discovered accidentally by a Polish-American chemist called Sternbach when in the course of clearing out his laboratory he came across a number of synthetic compounds for which no use had yet been found. Amongst them was chlordiazepoxide, which he sent for pharmacological tests on the off chance that it might have some useful and marketable properties. Sternbach's accidental discovery of chlordiazepoxide led to the biggest money-making bonanza in the entire history of medicine as a safe and universal 'cure-all' was launched into the sellers' market left by the barbiturate disaster. Chlordiazepoxide had been found to have sedating, muscle-relaxing, anticonvulsant and anti-aggressive properties. One writer noted that 'A taming effect was observed in rhesus monkeys, which can be very vicious in captivity.' Later, an advertisement for one of Librium's many chemical cousins was to bear a picture of a depressed housewife surrounded by mops, brooms and other tools of her trade, bearing the legend: 'You can't set her free, but you can help her feel less anxious.' As the benzodiazepine family multiplied and the competition in the marketplace hotted up, advertising became more and more blatant. The virtues of the pills were trumpeted in headlines, whilst their adverse effects were recorded in small print which would turn the writers of insurance policies green with envy. They were advertised as a solution to just about every problem known to man and suffered by women. Tensions between grandparents and grandchildren could now be cured by a pill. The anxieties suffered by a young woman leaving the family nest to go up to university could also be cured: 'A whole new world of anxiety . . . Her newly awakened intellectual curiosity may make her more anxious about international and domestic events.' Millions of pills were distributed free to doctors and teaching hospitals in order to establish competing brand names. All this added up to what must have been one of the most successful and profitable marketing exercises ever, and the promotion of the universal cure-all tranquillizer resulted in its becoming the most widely prescribed pill in the Western world. In 1986, some nine years after the peak of the sales of benzodiazepines, over 3,000 million Swiss francs of benzo-diazepine tranquillizers were sold worldwide.

Minor tranquillizers can be very useful drugs and are relatively safe when taken on their own. Then their side effects are usually less severe than those of other prescribed mood-altering drugs. But they have been and still are overused and overprescribed, and then their problems and hazards consider-ably outweigh their benefits. Minor tranquillizers are most often prescribed as sleeping tablets, which are often taken for years on end despite the fact that they don't actually work for more than two weeks at a time. When people have taken them for longer, they find that if they try to stop them they have difficulty in getting a good night's sleep. Whatever caused their insomnia in the first place, they now find it even more difficult to sleep because insomnia is a withdrawal effect of the pills. Thus, they are trapped in a vicious spiral of pill-taking. As a result they will be less alert, their memories will be less reliable, they will be more prone to accidents and to sudden explosions of rage or violent behaviour.

The use of pills to deal with insomnia more often than not obscures the real causes. Lack of exercise, too much coffee, irregular patterns of sleep, unresolved worries, boredom, grief and pain, all cause disturbances in sleep and none of these can be resolved by a pill. Elderly people in particular are likely to be prescribed sleeping pills and yet it is quite well known that after retirement people's life rhythms are disrupted. People get less exercise, the normal routines of working life are taken away, they may have catnaps during the day or fall asleep in front of television, so that when they go to bed they are unable to sleep. A great deal is known about sleep management, but unfortunately this knowledge is seldom put into practice in health services which are dominated by the prescription pad.

Women are prescribed minor tranquillizers three times more frequently than men and there has been a great deal of debate as to why this should be. It has been argued that this is a consequence of a male-dominated medical profession which sees women as being more emotional or more neurotic than men. Others say that women's lives are inherently more stressful than men's. The view that women should be constitu-tionally more prone to emotional disorders does not seem very logical and is not borne out by any systematic research. Why is it, for example, that single women tend to be more mentally healthy than married women, whilst married men tend to be more mentally healthy than single men? Does not evidence such as this point to social rather than physical factors determining the prescribing of tranquillizers? Many women's work consists of caring for their families and homes. Caring for children and dependent relatives may be infinitely more stressful than a man's work. However much men may complain about their jobs, those jobs offer them a clear and valued role, as well as a rich variety of experience. Caring for a demanding child or elderly relative is all the more stressful because it involves love and a degree of personal commitment far in excess of anything required by a job. What is more, women's work is not governed by the limits of the 35-hour week, or by the conditions set down by health and safety regulations. It is demanding in a way that no other work is demanding and it is often very isolating. Minor tranquillizers have been prescribed as the solution to these problems. But why? The use of these drugs defines those who take them as being sick and in need of medicine. It defines anxiety as a disease rather than as a healthy indication that something is wrong and requires action. For many people taking tranquillizers is akin to sitting on a fire and taking painkillers.

Benzodiazepine minor tranquillizers are labelled as either 'hypnotics' or 'anxiolytics', but there is little or no difference between them other than the length of their half-lives (i.e., the time it takes for the body to excrete half the active drug). A short-acting drug is active, therefore, for a shorter period of time than a long-acting one. A short-acting tranquillizer may be preferable to a long-acting one because it is less likely to cause a hangover the following day. In certain circumstances such differences may make one benzodiazepine more useful than another, but as far as any real distinctions between the differently labelled pills are concerned, they are as subtle as those between a brick and a half brick. Whatever the clever chemical manipulation of the basic compound, in the body most benzodiazepines are metabolized into the same basic active substances. The different names of these pills signify nothing more than a single product with many labels. In the following list of benzodiazepine tranquillizers, the different products are divided into hypnotics and anxiolytics, and then further divided into long- and short-acting compounds. The side and withdrawal effects are listed for the group as a whole.

Five-Point Guide to Getting the Most from Tranquillizers

For some people minor tranquillizers may be extremely useful as short-term aids to coping with a stressful event, but only if they are used wisely.

★ If you have been taking tranquillizers for more than two months, do not suddenly stop taking them – do it gradually, and preferably with the help of your doctor.

★ Use sleeping pills for as short a time as possible and remember that after between three and fourteen days your body has adjusted to them and they will no longer be helping you to sleep. If you are persistently unable to sleep you should consider whether your lifestyle and diet are causing your difficulties. If you must take them over long periods of time, do so intermittently. You will be doing your brain no good at all by embarking on a career of pill-taking.

★ Use anxiety-relieving pills for as short a time as possible and remember that they are more likely to have negative rather than positive effects on your life if you take them for too long. Ask yourself *why* you continue to feel anxious and whether you are really using the pills as a means for avoiding looking at what is really causing your anxiety. If you must take them, do so intermittently – use them as you would use an aspirin, that is, when you really must relieve a pain, and until you can get the cause of the pain looked at.

★ Don't listen to anyone who tells you that your insomnia or anxiety are caused by a chemical imbalance in your brain.

★ Minor tranquillizers should not be used to treat children except in very rare circumstances, such as night terrors.

Benzodiazepine Minor Tranquillizers

LONG-ACTING SLEEPING COMPOUNDS			
Generic name	*Trade name*	*Description*	*Dose*
Fluazepam	Dalmane	15 mg grey/ yellow capsules. 30 mg black/grey capsules.	15–30 mg per day.
	Paxane	15 mg green/grey capsules. 30 mg green/ black capsules.	
Flunitrazepam	Rohypnol	1 mg purple tablets.	0–5 – 1 mg per day.
Nitrazepam	Mogadon	5 mg purple/ black capsules.	5–10 mg per day.
	Somnite	Off-white liquid, to be taken orally.	
	Surem	5 mg mauve/grey capsules.	
	Under generic name	5 mg white tablets. Liquid to be taken orally.	

General Information

Long-acting drugs may be more likely to cause hangovers and have less severe withdrawal effects. Elderly and physically frail people should use half the above doses. These drugs can impair reflexes and the ability to drive a car.

SHORT-ACTING SLEEPING COMPOUNDS

Generic name	Trade name	Description	Dose
Loprazolam		1 mg white tablets.	Initially 1mg per day increased to 2.5–1.5 mg per day.
Lormeta-zepam		0.5 mg white tablets. 1 mg white tablets.	0.5–1.5 mg per day.
Temazepam		10 mg, 15 mg, 20 mg and 30 mg soft gelatin capsules. 10 mg and 20 mg hard gelatin capsules. 10 mg and 20 mg white tablets. Liquid to be taken orally.	10–30 mg, up to 40–60 mg per day.
Temazepam	Planpak	Cardboard box of pills with instructions.	Dose reduction pack for planned withdrawal from minor tranquillizers.
Triazolam	Halcion Under generic name	125 microgram lavender tablets. 250 microgram blue tablets. 125 and 250 microgram white tablets.	125–250 micro-grams per day.

General Information

Less likely than long-acting compounds to cause hangover but withdrawal effects may be more severe. Elderly and physically frail people should take half the above doses. These drugs can impair reflexes and the ability to drive a car.

LONG-ACTING ANXIETY COMPOUNDS

Generic name	Trade name	Description	Dose
Alprazolam	Xanax	250 microgram white tablets. 500 microgram pink tablets.	250–500 micrograms three times daily, increased if necessary to a total of 3 mg daily.
Bromezapam	Lexotan	1.5 mg lilac tablets. 3 mg pink tablets.	3–18 mg per day in divided doses. (In rate cases up to 60 mg per day may be given to hospital in-patients.)
Chlordiaze-poxide	Librium Under generic name	5 mg green/yellow capsules. 10 mg green/black capsules. 5 mg greenish-yellow tablets. 10 mg light-bluish-green tablets. 25 mg dark-bluish-green tablets. 5 mg, 10 mg and 25 mg white tablets. 5 mg and 10 capsules.	10 mg three times per day, increased if necessary to 60–100 mg per day.
Clobazam	Frisium Under generic name	10 mg hard gelatin capsules marked Frisium. 10 mg capsules marked s3B. (NB Marked s2B in Scotland.)	20–30 mg per day, up to a maximum dose of 60 mg per day in divided doses for hospital in-patients. For epilespsy, 20–30 mg per day, to a maximum of 60 mg per day. For children over three, the maximum dose is half the adult dose.

Generic name	Trade name	Description	Dose
Clorazepate dipotassium	Tranxene	7.5 mg maroon/grey capsules. 15 mg pink/grey capsules.	7.5–22.5 mg per day in divided doses.
Diazepam (NB there are a number of different branded forms of diazepam in injections and suppositories, but these are likely to be used in hospitals and dental surgeries and are not listed here.)	Valium	2 mg white tablets. 5 mg yellow tablets. 10 mg blue tablets. Pink syrup. Injection. Suppositories.	2 mg three times per day, increased if necessary to 15–30 mg daily in divided doses.) For children with nighttime terrors, 1–5 mg at bed-time.
	Under generic name	2 mg and 5 mg white tablets. Liquid to be taken orally.	
Medazepam	Nobrium	5 mg orange/yellow capsules. 10 mg orange/black capsules.	15–30 mg, increased if necessary to a maximum of 40 mg per day.

General Information

Withdrawal effects may be less severe than those of short-acting compounds. Elderly or physically frail people should receive half the adult dose. These drugs can impair reflexes and the ability to drive a car.

SHORT-ACTING ANXIETY COMPOUNDS

Generic name	Trade name	Description	Dose
Lorazepam	Ativan	1 mg blue tablets. 2.5 mg yellow tablets. Injection.	1–4 mg per day in divided doses.
Oxazepam	Oxanid	10 mg, 15 mg and 20 mg white tablets.	15–30 mg three to four times per day. For insomnia, 15–25 mg at bedtime (maximum dose 50 mg).
	Under generic name	30 mg capsules. 10 mg, 15 mg and 30 mg white tablets.	

General Information

Short-acting compounds may have more severe withdrawal effects than long-lasting ones. Withdrawal is best managed by switching to a long-acting compound for a planned gradual withdrawal. Elderly and physically frail people should use half the above doses. These drugs can impair reflexes and the ability to drive a car.

Benzodiazepine Minor Tranquillizers: Side Effects and Further Information

Common Side Effects

Feelings of tiredness, drowsiness and an inability to concentrate. Impairment of memory. Difficulty in co-ordinating movements. Ataxia (shaky movements and unsteady gait caused by the brain's failure to control the body's posture and the strength and direction of limb movements). Confusion (more likely in elderly people). Excitement, restlessness and aggressive behaviour.

Withdrawal

Withdrawal effects are: Anxiety. Insomnia. Agitation. Palpitations. 'Jelly legs'. Aches and pains. Restlessness. Panic attacks.

Sweating. Tremors. Pins and needles. Loss of appetite. Tension. Occasionally, convulsions.

How Benzodiazepines Interact with Other Drugs and Medicines

DRUG	Result of interaction
Alcohol	Increased sedation and increased intoxication.
Anaesthetics	Increased sedation.
Opioid painkillers such as codeine, pethidine, morphine	Increased sedation.
Erythromycin (an antibacterial drug)	Increases the blood level of triazolam.
Antidepressants	Increased sedation.
Anti-epileptic drugs	Reduces effect of clonazepam.
Antihistimines, for example common cold treatments, travel sickness pills, nasal inhalants, treatments for nettle rash	Increased sedation.
Drugs to reduce blood pressure	Increased reduction in blood pressure.
Antipsychotics	Increased sedation.
Disulfiram (a drug used to treat alcoholism)	Increased sedation with chlordiazepoxide and diazepam.
Levadopa (a drug used to treat Parkinsonism)	Benzodiazepines may reduce effectiveness of Levadopa.
Cimitadine (a drug used to treat ulcers)	Increased level of benzodiazepines in the blood stream.

that cannot be controlled or got rid of). Long-term psychotic illness, such as schizophrenia. Porphyria (a rare blood disorder which causes severe sensitivity to sunlight, resulting in inflammation or blistering of the skin, inflammation of the nerves, mental disturbances and attacks of stomach pain).

Conditions in which Benzodiazepines Should be Used with Caution

Respiratory disease. Muscle weakness. History of drug abuse. Pregnancy (particularly in the first three months). Breast-feeding. The elderly and physically frail should take reduced doses. Kidney and liver disease. Minor tranquillizers should not be taken over long periods of time.

Use in Pregnancy and Breast-feeding

There may be a very small chance of a baby being born with a cleft palate if the mother is taking a benzodiazepine during the first three months of her pregnancy. Children of mothers taking benzodiazepines have been born suffering from the 'floppy baby syndrome', a condition in which the child is withdrawn, drowsy, listless and seemingly indifferent to feeding. This condition improves once the drug has been excreted from the baby's system. If the mother has taken them throughout her pregnancy, there is the risk that a newly born child could be exposed to the withdrawal effects. The drugs also pass from mother to infant in the breast milk, which can cause weight loss and lethargy in the baby. The long-term effects of a mother's chronic use of benzodiazepines during pregnancy on her unborn child's development have never been monitored.

Elderly People and Benzodiazepines

As we grow older our bodily functions slow down, which often means that any drugs we consume will remain in our bodies for longer. In some circumstances this may not be a problem, but in others it can cause serious complications. There have been a number of scandals in old people's homes involving the overdrugging, whether by accident or design, of residents. The quality of prescribing in old people's homes in the recent past has been shown to leave much to be desired. As benzodiazepines may take much longer than normal to leave an elderly person's system, the regular use of tranquillizers can result in the amount of the drug being gradually built up to dangerous levels. When taking these drugs elderly people may also be much more prone to falls resulting in serious injuries. Concern about this type of accident has been voiced in the medical press by orthopaedic surgeons. Elderly people are more vulnerable to suffering from the side effects of drugs and great caution is required in the way that drugs are prescribed and administered.

As well as benzodiazepines, there are several other minor tranquillizers which are prescribed for the treatment of anxiety and insomnia. Their properties and effects are listed below.

Over Anxiety-relieving Drugs

BUSPIRONE

Trade name	Ingredients
Buspar	5 mg white tablets engraved with 5. 10 mg white tablets engraved with 10.

General Information

Buspirone is a relatively new drug for the treatment of anxiety, having been in use in Britain since 1985. In these circumstances it may be some time before we know how valuable buspirone really is. It appears to have a number of advantages over the benzodiazepines, as well as a few disadvantages. It is said that buspirone does not cause sedation or physical dependence, impair physical skills or co-ordination, and that it is safe in overdose. The major disadvantage it appears to have is that it may take up to four weeks before it relieves anxiety. As it does not cause sedation, buspirone has no place in the treatment of insomnia. How the drug exerts its effects is unknown. Like all the drugs in this group, it can impair reflexes and the ability to drive a car.

Dosage Information

Adult (16 and over): Treatment begins with 5 mg two to three times daily, which may be increased if necessary every two or three days to the usual dose range of between 15–30 mg per day. **The maximum dose is 45 mg per day.**

Elderly and physically frail: The maximum dose for elderly people is 30 mg per day.

Side Effects and Further Information

The side effects of buspirone are said to become less severe with time. If side effects do become a problem, the manufacturers recommend a reduction in dose. According to the manufacturers, 'the only side effects that occurred with significantly greater frequency with buspirone treatment than with a placebo were dizziness, headaches, nervousness, light-headedness, excitement and nausea. Tachycardia (increased heart rate), palpitations, chest pain, drowsiness, confusion, dry mouth, fatigue, sweating and clamminess have also been reported rarely.'

Conditions in which Buspirone Must be Avoided

Epilepsy. Severe liver or kidney disease. Pregnancy and breast-feeding. It should not be used concurrently with MAOI (Monoamine oxidase inhibitor) antidepressants.

Conditions in which Buspirone Should be Used with Caution

When there is a history of liver or kidney disease. Buspirone is of no use in the treatment of the withdrawal effects of benzodiazepines.

CHLORMEZANONE	
Trade name	*Ingredients*
Trancopal	200 mg yellow tablets.

General Information

Chlormezanone is a mildly sedating compound which may be used for the short-term treatment of anxiety, insomnia and muscle spasms. It may be prescribed with painkillers to relieve conditions like arthritis. It is a sedating drug which may cause drowsiness. When used for sleep disorders it may have a hangover effect of drowsiness the following day. It can also impair reflexes and the ability to drive a car.

Dosage Information

Adult (16 and over): 200 mg three to four times per day, or 400 mg in a single dose at bedtime.

Elderly and physically frail: Elderly people should take half the adult dose.

Side Effects and Further Information

Drowsiness and lethargy. Dizziness. Nausea. Headache. Dry mouth. Rashes. Jaundice. If used for more than a few weeks dependency can occur.

Conditions in which Chlormezanone Must be Avoided

Serious lung disorders. Depressed breathing. Porphyria (a rare blood disorder which causes severe sensitivity to sunlight, resulting in inflammation or blistering of the skin, inflammation of the nerves, mental disturbances and attacks of stomach pain).

Conditions in which Chlormezanone Should be Used with Caution

Respiratory disease. Where there is a history of drug dependency. Muscular weakness. Pregnancy and breast-feeding (see below). The elderly and physically frail should receive reduced doses. It should only be used for short-term treatment and should be withdrawn gradually.

Use in Pregnancy and Breast-feeding

There are no reports of damage to the unborn child but if the mother takes this drug for long periods of time during pregnancy, the foetus will be exposed to sedation and the risk of dependence which could lead to the new-born baby experiencing withdrawal effects.

HYDROXYZINE

Trade name	Ingredients
Atarax	10 mg orange tablets. 25 mg green tablets. Syrup to be taken orally.

General Information

Hydroxyzine is used for the short-term relief of anxiety and insomnia. It may also be used to enhance the effect of painkillers and in the treatment of asthma. Rather unusually for this group of drugs, hydroxyzine is said to have little potential for causing dependence. Like all the drugs in this group, however, it can impair reflexes and the ability to drive a car. Some patients may be sensitive to this drug.

Dosage Information

Adult (16 and over): 50–100 mg per day.

Adult and physically frail: The elderly and physically frail should receive a lower dose.

Side Effects and Further Information

The side effects of hydroxyzine are said to be mild and infrequent. The most commonly reported side effects are disturbances of vision, drowsiness and itching.

Conditions in which Hydroxyzine Must be Avoided

Sensitivity to hydroxyzine. Pregnancy (see below).

Conditions in which Hydroxyzine Should be Used with Caution

Caution should be exercised in using the drug concurrently with barbiturates, alcohol, opiates and other tranquillizers.

Use in Pregnancy and Breast-feeding

Avoid using in pregnancy, particularly during the first three months. Studies in animals have shown risks to the foetus but these have not been confirmed in humans. Nevertheless, as with all sedating drugs, there is a risk that the unborn and newly born may be affected.

MEPROBROMATE

Trade name	Description
Equagesic	Three-layered tablets, a white layer sandwiched between pink and yellow layers. The tablets contain 75 mg ethoheptazine, 150 mg meprobromate and 250 mg aspirin.
Equanil	200 mg white tablets. 400 mg white tablets.
Tenavoid	200 mg meprobromate plus 3 mg bendrofluazide orange tablets.

General Information

Meprobromate is less effective as a tranquillizer than the benzodiazepines, is more dangerous in overdose, more likely to cause dependence and has more severe withdrawal effects. Tenavoid is a combination of meprobromate and a diuretic and its manufacturers promote it as a treatment for premenstrual tension, but is not recommended for use by the British National Formulary. Equagesic is an altogether extraordinary mixture of two painkillers, aspirin, ethoheptazine and meprobromate, and its manufacturers promote it as a short-term treatment for 'the symptomatic relief of pain occurring in musculo-skeletal disorders.' Equagesic does not rate a mention in the BNF and it is perhaps a matter of concern that such a potentially dangerous compound should be presented in a form of pill that looks so much like a sherbet sweet. Meprobromate may have some uses but it is difficult to see what these may be, given the very many other less hazardous compounds available in this group.

Dosage Information

Adult (16 and over): 400 mg three to four times a day.

Elderly and physically frail: Elderly people should receive half the adult dose or less.

Side Effects and Further Information

Meprobromate has a wide range of side effects and these are more frequent and more hazardous than those of the benzodiazepine group. It is also potentially addictive as tolerance develops rapidly, which means that increased doses may be required to achieve the drug's marginal benefits. If the drug is used over any length of time the patient may develop a craving for it. The withdrawal effects of mebrobromate are: Drowsiness, Light-headedness. Confusion. Ataxia (shaky movements and unsteady gait caused by the brain's failure to control the body's posture and the strength and direction of limb movements). Impaired memory. Headaches. Vertigo. Dry mouth. Stomach upsets. Reduced urination. Agranulocytosis (a serious deficiency of white blood cells caused by damage to the bone marrow). Allergic reactions. Convulsions. Paradoxically, excitement. Paraesthesia (pins and needles). Tolerance to the effects of drug. Addiction.

Withdrawal

Not every patient experiences withdrawal effects, but many do. The effects may be sufficiently severe to be life-threatening if left untreated. The effects are: Anxiety. Feelings of weakness. Tension. Loss of appetite. Epileptic fits. Delirium. Hallucinations. Sudden withdrawal may cause fits.

Conditions in which Meprobromate Must be Avoided

Severe lung and breathing problems. Pregnancy and breast-feeding. Porphyria (a rare blood disorder which causes severe sensitivity to sunlight, resulting in inflammation or blistering of the skin, inflammaton of the nerves, mental disturbances and attacks of stomach pain). Meprobromate should only be used when no alternative treatment is available.

Conditions in which Meprobromate Should be Used with Caution

Epilepsy (meprobromate may cause fits). Respiratory disease. History of drug dependence. Pregnancy. Kidney and liver disease.

Use in Pregnancy and Breast-feeding

Avoid completely.

The Barbiturates

In treatment of anxiety or insomnia there is no place for any of the barbiturate compounds, except for a diminishing number of elderly people who have been maintained on them for many years. The only reason that such patients are maintained on these highly dangerous drugs is the fact that it would be too difficult or too dangerous to wean them off. Despite the fact the number of prescriptions for barbiturates has steadily declined over the past 30 years, they continue to cause a large proportion of the deaths from overdose or suicide recorded in Britain. Barbiturates are more dangerous than heroin, as they have worse side effects and withdrawal effects, and are considerably more difficult and hazardous to withdraw from. Withdrawal from barbiturates can be fatal. They do have a small but problematical role in the control of epilepsy and in anaesthesia, but apart from these their only, and somewhat dubious, distinction is that of being the drug of choice for suicide, for which they are extremely effective. It is extremely unlikely that any doctor will prescribe barbiturates for anxiety or insomnia to a patient not already hooked on them, and any who do should be avoided like a plague.

BARBITURATE PRODUCTS

Trade name	Description
Amytal	30 mg white tablets marked T56. 50 mg white tablets marked T37. 100 mg white tablets marked T32. 200 mg white tablets marked U13
Seconal Sodium	50 mg orange capsules marked F42. 100 mg orange capsules marked F40.
Sodium Amytal	60 mg blue capsules marked F23. 60 mg white tablets marked U43. 200 mg blue capsules marked F33. 200 mg white tablets marked U16.
Soneryl	100 mg pink tablets.
Tuinal	100 mg orange/blue capsules marked F65.

General Information

Barbiturates should only be prescribed to patients who have been treated with them for a considerable length of time and for whom it is impossible to stop prescribing them because of the risks associated with withdrawal. In effect, they are now used for the maintenance of addicted patients. These compounds are controlled under the provisions of the Misuse of Drugs Regulations, 1985.

Dosage Information

Amytal: 100–200 mg at bedtime.
Seconal Sodium: 50–100 mg at bedtime.
Sodium Amytal: 60–200 mg at bedtime.
Soneryl: 100–200 mg at bedtime.
Tuinal: 100–200 mg at bedtime.

Side effects and Further Information

Elderly people are particularly vulnerable to the side effects of these drugs, but at the same time they are more likely to be taking them than anyone else, apart from addicts, amongst whom they are very popular. Elderly people metabolize drugs much more slowly than younger people do, which can lead to the drug building up in their bodies to dangerous and potentially fatal levels. Side effects include: Drowsiness. Lightheadedness. Confusion. Ataxia (shaky movements and unsteady gait caused by the brain's failure to control the body's posture and the strength and direction of limb movements). Impaired memory. Headaches. Vertigo. Dry mouth. Stomach upsets. Reduced urination. Agranulocytosis (a serious deficiency of white blood cells caused by damage to the bone marrow). Allergic reactions. Convulsions. Paradoxical, excitement. Paraesthesia (pins and needles). Tolerance to the effects of the drug. Addiction.

Withdrawal

The withdrawal effects of barbiturate compounds may be sufficiently severe to be life-threatening if left untreated. The effects are: Anxiety. Feelings of weakness. Tension. Loss of appetite. Epileptic fits. Delirium. Hallucinations. According to a standard psychiatric textbook by Slater and Roth (1969), when barbiturates were withdrawn after chronic intoxication 'an acute withdrawal psychosis clinically resembling delirium tremens with anxiety and terrifying hallucinations, occurred in three out of five cases, two or three days after admission to hospital.'

Conditions in which Barbiturates Must be Avoided

Barbiturates should not be used at all for anxiety and insomnia, but they are even more dangerous in the following conditions: Porphyria (a rare blood disorder which causes severe sensitivity to sunlight resulting in inflammation or blistering of the skin, inflammation of the nerves, mental disturbances and attacks of stomach pain). Insomnia caused by pain.

Use in Pregnancy and Breast-Feeding

Avoid completely.

Other Insomnia-relieving Products

CHLORAL HYDRATE	
Trade name	Description
Chloral mixture	Foul-tasting liquid, to be diluted and taken orally.
Chloral elixir, Paediatric	Foul-tasting liquid with blackcurrant flavour, to be diluted and taken orally.
Welldorm	Bluish-purple capsule containing 707 mg choral betaine, which is the equivalent of 414 mg of chloral hydrate. Foul-tasting liquid with passion-fruit flavour, to be diluted and taken orally.

General Information

The use in psychiatry of chloral hydrate goes back to the last century; it is mentioned in a psychiatric textbook written in 1899 by Emil Kraepelin, one of the leading pioneers of modern psychiatry. His brief entry on the drug reads: 'Chloral hydrate: Induces longer sleep, sometimes with drowsiness in the morning. Mordant, unpleasant taste.' It does indeed have an extremely bitter and unpleasant taste which is barely concealed by the fruit flavours added to make it more palatable. If it comes into contact with the skin it can cause irritation.

Chloral hydrate is used in the short-term treatment of insomnia. The treatment of insomnia in children by drugs is controversial, but if it is necessary the treatment should not be given for longer than one or two days at a time. If the problem persists it is wise to seek non-medical methods of treatment. Behaviour therapy has been successfully used to treat sleeping difficulties in infants and children. Quite often insomnia in children can be traced to anxieties caused by difficulties being experienced by their parents. In such circumstances the use of drugs not only fails to address the underlying anxieties causing the insomnia, but unnecessarily exposes the child to the hazards of drugs. In comparison with other drugs used to treat insomnia, chloral hydrate is relatively safe, but in long-term use it can lead to dependence and addiction. Ideally, drugs should be used as the very last resort for the treatment of insomnia, particularly for children.

Dosage Information

Adult (16 and over): *Chloral mixture*: 5–20 ml taken 15 to 30 minutes before bedtime.

Noctec: 500 mg–1g.

Welldorm capsules: One to two capsules at bedtime.

Welldorm elixir: 15–45 ml taken 15 to 30 minutes before bedtime.

The maximum daily dose is 2g with plenty of water.

Elderly and physically frail: Should receive same doses as for adults.

Children: *Chloral mixture*: For children aged one to five, 2.5–5 ml; aged six to twelve, 5–10 ml, taken 15 to 30 minutes before bedtime.

Choral elixir (paediatric): For children up to one year old, 5 ml, well diluted.

Noctec: Not recommended for children.

Welldorm capsules and elixir: Doses are calculated by body weight: 30–50 mg and 1–1.7 ml per kilogram of body weight.

The maximum single dose is 1g per day, to be taken in with plenty of water.

Side Effects and Further Information

Chloral hydrate quite commonly causes stomach upsets. Although rare, it can also cause rashes, headache, ketonuria (the presence of acetone in the urine), excitement and delirium. Long-term use may cause kidney damage and dependence. Avoid contact with skin. Avoid long-term use and abrupt withdrawal.

Conditions in which Chloral Hydrate Must Be Avoided

Severe heart disease. Upset stomach. Serious liver or kidney disease.

Conditions in which Chloral Hydrate Should Be Used with Caution

Where there is a history of drug dependence. Pregnancy and breast-feeding (see below). Lung or respiratory disease.

Use in Pregnancy and Breast-feeding

Like other drugs chloral hydrate passes from the mother to the foetus in the womb and from the mother to the newly born child through breast milk. In the unlikely event that a mother takes chloral hydrate for prolonged periods during pregnancy the unborn child will be exposed to all of the effects listed above.

TRICLOFOS	
Trade name	*Description*
Triclofos Elixir	Liquid to be taken 30 minutes before bedtime.

General Information

Triclofos is a derivative of chloral hydrate and has similar effects, although it is less likely to cause stomach ulcers. For details of effects and side effects, see the above entry for chloral hydrate.

Dosage Information

Adult (16 and over): 1–2g 30 minutes before bedtime. Max dose = 2g

Elderly and physically frail: The elderly and physically frail should receive reduced doses.

Children: For children up to 1 year of age, 100–250 mg; between one and five years old, 250–500 mg; and between six and twelve years old, 500 mg–1g.

Depression

We use the word depressed to convey to others that we feel sad or unhappy. We may be depressed about losing a job, because of a bereavement or as a consequence of any distressing event in our lives, although sometimes we feel depressed for no obvious reason. (Winston Churchill called the bouts of depression he suffered throughout his adult life his 'black dog'.) But when do these emotions amount to a depression meriting treatment? The simple answer is when extreme sadness, pessimism or despair dominate a person's consciousness and behaviour for an intolerable period of time. Most people recover from their depression with time and the help of those around them, but some seem to sink still further into despair. When this happens and they seek the help of their doctors they are likely to be diagnosed as depressed.

Some people are diagnosed as suffering 'reactive' depression, meaning that it is a reaction to distressing circumstances, others as suffering from 'endogenous' depression, that is, their depression appears not to have any external cause and is thus assumed to come from within the sufferer. Not everyone agrees that it is useful or even possible to draw such distinctions, although some drug manufacturers claim that their products are particularly beneficial for one or other of these categories.

Clinical Depression

Depression becomes 'clinical' when it has been diagnosed as such by a doctor. 'Clinical depression' is not a specific illness but a term used for a set of symptoms and signs which doctors judge to be serious enough to require treatment. As for the actual causes of these symptoms, however, the term 'clinical' adds little to our understanding of them. There are many theories about the nature and causes of depression and although research points to some convincing factors, there is no one cause. It is not something that can be caught, like influenza or chickenpox, and neither is it caused by delinquent brain cells or genes, although in some circumstances these may play a part. Depression is the culmination of changes occurring in the mind, body and life of the sufferer. It can be effectively relieved by drugs, but there is no drug which cures it. The good news is that about 60 per cent of people who suffer depression get better, with or without treatment.

Symptoms or Signs of 'Clinical' Depression

Changes in Mood: Feelings of gloom and pessimism. Feelings of sadness which are impossible to shake off. A deep sense of personal isolation – feeling cut off from surroundings and other people. These feelings are usually more intense early in the morning or late at night.

Guilt: Nagging feelings of guilt, worthlessness and shame. Sometimes very severely depressed people develop strange ideas and fixed beliefs about themselves or others to the point where they lose contact with reality. They may see, hear, smell or feel touched by things that are not really there. This may be called psychotic depression.

Problems with sleep: Difficulty in getting off to sleep because of persistent fears and anxiety. Sleep becomes fitful, with bouts of restlessness and agitation. Waking up very early in the morning feeling anxious, unrested and drained.

Problems with work and activities: Feeling increasingly unable to cope with the daily demands of work. Continual anxiety, leading to increasing difficulties in making even the simplest decisions and feeling plagued by doubt over any decision made. Everything seems to require more and more effort and less seems to be achieved or achievable. Loss of interest and loss of will. This may lead to a gradual withdrawal from daily activities and contact with other people.

Agitation and anxiety: Anxiety becomes persistent, which may lead to agitation and explosions of rage which are often followed by bouts of extreme remorse.

Slowing down: Thought processes become sluggish and concentration becomes increasingly difficult. The limbs and body feel heavier and require more effort to move. Memory becomes less reliable. Feeling apathetic and increasingly driven inward into the self.

Morbid thoughts and ideas: Obsessive concern or preoccupation with physical health. Minor aches and pains become major worries. Sometimes a fixed belief in an undiagnosed illness. Feelings of unreality, detachment and isolation.

Physical signs and symptoms: Indigestion, wind, constipation, loss of appetite and feelings of heaviness in the stomach. Headaches. Palpitations or heart flutters. Overbreathing. Backache. Muscular aches and pains. Lethargy and persistent fatigue.

Also, reduced sexual arousal, premature ejaculation, impotence, inability to reach orgasm. Periods may become irregular, occurring more or less frequently than usual. Period pains may be more severe and the period heavier.

Loss of weight.

Suicidal tendencies: A preoccupation with suicidal thoughts, ideas and speculations which may be acted upon.

Each year more than eight million prescriptions for antidepressants are dispensed in Britain. Estimates as to the proportion of adults in the population diagnosed as clinically depressed vary between two and fifteen per hundred. The large gap between these lower and higher estimates is explained in part by the fact that some doctors are more likely to diagnose it than others. Studies have shown a social-class bias in the way that depression is diagnosed, with middle-class people more likely to be diagnosed as suffering from anxiety or stress, and working-class people more likely to be diagnosed as depressed.

One very striking feature about depression is the fact that women are twice as likely as men to be diagnosed as depressed. The difference in the rates cannot be explained by hormonal or other gender-related physical factors. Premenstrual problems, postnatal depression and the menopause, play very small parts in the overall figures.

A gender-related difference which may help to explain women's increased likelihood of suffering depression is the different ways in which the sexes deal with emotional distress. Men are twice as likely as women to become alcoholic or drug abusers, a type of behaviour which may represent a form of 'self-medication'. Such an explanation fits very neatly with the finding that women are more likely than men to seek help from their doctors. Thus, while men are more likely to be seen in the pub when they are low, women are more likely to be seen in the GP's waiting room. Men are substantially more prone to committing crimes, particularly violent crimes. Again, this fits with the view that men tend to externalize their feelings through aggressive behaviour, whilst women tend to internalize them by becoming anxious or depressed.

A broader, socio-economic perspective may also shed some light on women's apparent increased vulnerability to depression. One of the key features of the experience of depression is a feeling of powerlessness. An interesting recent research finding which may have some bearing here is one which suggests that people who are prone to depression are more likely to have a realistic view of life than those who do not. And in a world in which patriarchy in its many forms is prevalent, the objective reality is that women exercise less power in society than men.

A research study done amongst women in Camberwell, South London, showed that about a quarter of working-class women living with children suffered from depression. Amongst these a large proportion would have been diagnosed by a doctor as suffering from depression serious enough to warrant medication or admission to hospital. The rate amongst middle-class women in the same area was 6 per cent. Of the depressed working-class women, most had experienced a serious problem in the previous year, such as the loss of a husband or serious financial problems. However, research into problems such as depression seldom includes the broader socio-economic issues which have such a bearing on the lives of the subjects of that research. Much of it focuses narrowly on personal problems or responses to treatment with drugs. One of the great difficulties of research into mental health is that it seldom looks at the world in which mental ill health occurs. But perhaps there is a risk that we might discover things that we would rather not know about?

Tricyclic Antidepressants

The term tricyclic refers to the molecular structure of these drugs which comprises three linked rings of molecules, although not all the antidepressants which are usually classified as tricyclics have this structure. Some are in fact 'bicyclics', whilst others are 'tetracyclics' or 'monocyclics'. The actual distinctions between them are relatively unimportant, however, as regardless of the way the ingredients are combined, in their effects and side effects, most of these drugs have more similarities than differences. Despite the claims made for these products by their manufacturers, which influence the way doctors prescribe them, the practical differences between them is of little more importance to the consumer than the differences between competing brands of petrol, washing powder or baked beans.

The first of the tricyclic antidepressants was imipramine, which was introduced in 1957 and was followed soon after by amitriptyline. Since then many new products have been added to the tricyclic group, although it appears that doctors maintain some degree of scepticism about the advantages claimed for the newer or 'second-generation' tricyclic antidepressants. Amitriptyline and imipramine remain the most widely prescribed drugs in the group, accounting for just under two-thirds of all prescriptions for antidepressants drugs in Britain. Apart from the fact that these older drugs are as good as more recent ones, they have the added advantage of being considerably less expensive to our beleaguered National Health Service.

How Effective are Tricyclic Antidepressants?

Tricyclic antidepressants are effective in reducing the symptoms of depression and can therefore make life more bearable for many people. But they do not work for everyone, and little is actually known about how or why they work. Between 65 and 70 per cent of people who have been diagnosed as suffering from depression can expect to feel less depressed within two to four weeks of starting treatment with a tricyclic antidepressant. Thirty per cent, however, will feel better if they are given a placebo, that is, a dummy drug with no active ingredients whatsoever and possibly containing nothing more potent than chalk or sugar. A review of the controlled studies into the effectiveness of tricyclic antidepressants reveals that more than a third of all such studies showed the active drugs to have been no more effective than the placebos. Nevertheless, whatever the scientific facts, the truth is that many thousands of depressed people feel less depressed when they take them. Whether and to what extent this improvement is due to what medical researchers call the 'placebo effect', or even to old-fashioned magic, is less important than the fact that for many people these drugs are the only means available to them to relieve the misery of their depression.

Side Effects – A Cause For Concern

All medicines have their disadvantages and side effects. The old saying 'No pain no gain', despite its puritan echoes, is well borne in mind when considering treatment with antidepressants. The side effects of antidepressant drugs can be, and often are, severe, so much so that less than half of all prescribed antidepressants are actually taken. Most of them are either thrown away or abandoned in medicine cabinets as dangerous, half-forgotten hoards. When asked, the main reason people give for not persevering with their treatment is that they find the side effects of antidepressants intolerable. These can be particularly severe during the early stages of treatment, before any benefit is felt from taking the drug. It can take up to four weeks before the symptoms of the depression are reduced, and during this time many people will feel worse and often more depressed than they did before they started taking the drug. In these circumstances it is not surprising that so many simply stop taking them. However, the combination of the early side effects and the late benefits of these drugs can have tragic consequences.

In Britain at least 300 people take their lives each year using a tricyclic antidepressant, often in combination with tranquillizers or alcohol. It is easy to assume that because those concerned were depressed their deaths were simply the consequences of an illness called depression. It is just as easy to forget that the people who take their lives with these drugs obtain them from their doctors in lethal quantities. Their deaths raise serious issues concerning the quality of care available to people in serious mental distress.

The massive over-prescription of benzodiazepines like

Valium, Ativan and Mogadon also points towards major problems in the quality of our mental health services. For example, in Britain the average length of a consultation with a general practitioner is said to be six and a half minutes; the average length of a consultation with a psychiatrist, ten minutes.

A survey done by MIND and the BBC *That's Life!* programme amongst more than two thousand long-term tranquillizer users revealed that over 77 per cent had seen their doctors for less than 15 minutes when they were first prescribed tranquillizers. Sixty-eight per cent were not given any information about the drugs being prescribed. Less than half were told they were being prescribed a tranquillizer. Over 47 per cent of those surveyed had received treatment from a psychiatric hospital and of those two-thirds described their psychiatric treatment as being of no help or as being positively harmful. At the time of their first prescriptions a quarter of the survey were given prescriptions for more than one mood-altering drug; by the time they received their sixth the proportion of people prescribed more than one mood-altering drug had risen to half the sample.

The majority of people with serious depression who seek the help of their doctors will be offered a prescription for a tricyclic antidepressant. Some will take the drug as an important part of an individually tailored treatment programme which they regularly review with their doctor. In these circumstances the drugs are most likely to be effective. Many people, however, will get little more than repeat prescriptions for the drugs for as long as they continue to collect them. In these circumstances the real value of the tricyclic antidepressants must be questionable.

Getting the Most from Tricyclic Antidepressants

Depression is a life-diminishing and sometimes a life-threatening condition. The decision to begin a course of medical treatment should be regarded as a major life event for the individual, the family and those closest to him or her. Quite often when a person is seriously depressed he or she is unable or reluctant to consider the pros and cons of embarking on a course of treatment and in such circumstances a husband, wife or friend may wish to share in the decision-making process. In order for that process to be meaningful it must be as informed as possible. A knowledge of side effects may be of crucial importance to all concerned. Those around the depressed person may need to reassure him or her that any strange new feelings and discomforts are caused by the drug rather than by a deterioration of his or her mental state. They may also wish to reassure him or her that these side effects may become less troublesome and that some relief can be expected in time. If the drug does not bring relief within an acceptable period, about eight weeks, they may support the individual in seeking an alternative form of treatment. When the time comes to stop taking it they may give help and support during the withdrawal period.

Eight-Point Guide to Getting the Most from Tricyclic Antidepressants

★ Tricyclic antidepressants do not cure depression but they do provide effective relief from most of it symptoms for most people who have them appropriately prescribed. A significant minority – between 30 and 40 per cent will obtain no benefit from them.

★ The side effects of this group of drugs can be severe, particularly at the outset of treatment and until they begin to diminish the feelings of depression.

★ All antidepressants are extremely dangerous in overdose.

★ It is important that tricyclic drugs are taken as and when they are prescribed. In some circumstances it is advisable that someone close to the depressed person take charge of the medication, rather than leaving the person with large quantities of pills.

★ The need for the antidepressant to be continued should be reviewed with the doctor at least every six months.

★ Whilst tricyclic antidepressants are not addictive they do have withdrawal effects. If the antidepressant has been taken for more than a few days the drug should not be suddenly stopped but the dose should be gradually reduced over a period of at least 12 weeks.

★ Most depressed people get better with time with or without treatment.

★ Treatment with drugs can be an important step towards eventual recovery but *it is equally important that the social and emotional circumstances in which the person became depressed be reviewed and possibly changed to achieve a lasting recovery.*

FAST FACTS	Tricyclic Antidepressants
Purpose	Treatment of depression.
How do I take it?	Tablets or syrup.
When do I take it?	As directed by your doctor.
How long does it take to work?	Between two and four weeks.
Should I expect to experience side effects?	Yes. particularly when you first start taking the drug, but many people find that they become less troublesome as time passes.
What are the most common side effects?	Dry mouth; tiredness; reduced sexual feelings; less frequent urination; constipation; blurred vision; trembling hands; increased appetite; a craving for sweet foods.
What should I do if I experience other distressing side effects?	Notify your doctor.
How long should I continue to take the drug?	This will depend on your needs and circumstances but at least every six months you should review the need to continue with the drug with your doctor.
Is it addictive?	No, but if you have taken the antidepressant for more than a month you may experience withdrawal effects. You should withdraw from this drug by a gradual reduction in the dose taken over a period of eight weeks.
Can I drive whilst taking it?	Antidepressants will affect your ability to drive safely.
Can I drink alcohol whilst taking it?	If you drink alcohol it will interact with the drug and further impair your ability to drive. It may make you feel ill.

NEVER EXCEED THE PRESCRIBED DOSE · ALWAYS INFORM ANY DENTIST, DOCTOR OR ANAESTHETIST WHO TREATS YOU THAT YOU ARE TAKING THIS DRUG · KEEP MEDICINES OUT OF THE REACH OF CHILDREN

AMITRIPTYLINE

Trade name	Description
Amitriptyline Hydrochloride	Injection.
Domical	10 mg blue tablets. 25 mg orange tablets. 50 mg red-brown tablets.
Lentizol	25 mg pink capsules. 50 mg pink and red capsules.
Tryptizol	10 mg blue tablets. 25 mg yellow tablets. 50 mg brown tablets. Pink syrup to be drunk as directed by doctor or pharmacist.

General Information

One of the first and most commonly prescribed tricyclic antidepressants. Effective for the treatment of depression in about 65 to 70 per cent of people who have been correctly diagnosed. It takes between two and four weeks before the antidepressant effects are felt.

Dosage Information

Adult (16 and over): Treatment begins with 50–75 mg daily in divided doses or preferably in a single dose at bedtime, increased gradually if necessary to **a maximum of 150–200 mg per day**. The usual maintenance dose is 50–100 mg per day.

Elderly, physically frail and adolescent: Initially 25–50 mg, increased with caution and close medical supervision to **a maximum of 150 mg per day**.

Children: Amitriptyline is not recommended for the treatment of depression in children below the age of 16. Amitriptyline causes urinary retention and for this reason is sometimes used as a treatment for bedwetting in children. Not everyone agrees that this is an appropriate way to deal with the problems of children who wet the bed.

Dose of Amitriptyline Used in the Treatment of Bedwetting	
Age of child and body weight	*Daily dose*
6–10 years (20–35 kg/44–77 lbs) 11–16 years (35–54 kg/77–119 lbs)	10–20 mg. 25–50 mg

The dose appropriate for the age and body weight of the child should *not* be exceeded. Treatment should not exceed a period of three months, *including* a period of gradual withdrawal from the drug. The bedwetting may return when the drug is withdrawn. However, treatment with antidepressants should not be resumed without a thorough physical examination of the child or in circumstances where other forms of help such as child guidance, counselling or psychological methods have not been attempted. The treatment of bedwetting with antidepressants should be regarded as a last resort.

> **OVERDOSE EXTREMELY DANGEROUS · SEEK IMMEDIATE MEDICAL HELP**

Side Effects and Further Information

See pp. 70–73.

AMOXAPINE

Trade name	Description
Asendis	25 mg white hexagonal tablets marked LL25. 50 mg orange hexagonal tablets marked LL50. 100 mg blue hexagonal tablets marked LL100. 150 mg white hexagonal tablets marked LL150.

General Information

Amoxapine is closely related to the so-called major tranquillizers and has similar effects and side effects to other tricyclic antidepressants. It can relieve the symptoms of depression within four to seven days of beginning the treatment, as compared to many tricyclic antidepressants which can take between two and four weeks to bring relief. Until the benefits of the drug begin to be felt side effects may cause more problems and the depression may grow worse.

Dosage Information

Adult (16 and over): Initially 100–150 mg daily in divided doses or, preferably, in a single dose at bedtime, to be increased gradually if necessary to **a maximum of 300 mg daily**. The usual maintenance dose is 150–250 mg per day.

Elderly and physically frail: Treatment begins with 25 mg twice daily, to be increased if necessary after five to seven days to **a maximum of 50 mg three times daily**.

Children: Amoxapine is not recommended for children.

OVERDOSE EXTREMELY DANGEROUS · SEEK IMMEDIATE
MEDICAL HELP

Side Effects and Further Information

Women may experience irregular periods and milk may be secreted from their breasts. In long-term use there is a risk of developing a condition called tardive dyskinesia which causes involuntary movements in the mouth, face, trunk and limbs. This condition may be permanent. For a fuller description and discussion of tardive dyskinesia, see p. 160–162.

For further information, see pp. 70–73.

BUTRIPTYLINE

Trade name	Description
Evadyne	25 mg orange tablets.

General Information

One of the newer tricyclic antidepressants whose effects and side effects are similar to those of amitriptyline. It is claimed that butriptyline is less sedating than other drugs in this group. It may take between two and four weeks before the symptoms of depression are relieved. During this time the side effects may cause more problems and the feelings of depression grow worse.

Dosage Information

Adult (16 and over): Treatment begins with 25 mg three times daily, to be increased gradually if necessary to **a maximum of 150 mg**. The usual maintenance dose is 25 mg three times daily.

Elderly and physically frail: The elderly and physically frail should receive reduced doses.

Children: Not recommended for the treatment of children.

Side Effects and Further Information

See pp. 70–73.

CLOMIPRAMINE	
Trade name	*Description*
Anafranil	10 mg yellow and brown capsules. 25 mg orange and brown capsules. 50 mg blue and brown capsules. 75 mg pink tablets. Orange-coloured and -flavoured syrup to be taken as directed by doctor or chemist. Injection.
Clomipramine (generic name)	10 mg tablets. 25 mg tablets. 50 mg tablets.

General Information

Clomipramine is similar in its effects and side effects to other tricyclic antidepressants and thus probably has no obvious benefits or disadvantages over such drugs as amitriptyline. It is claimed to have benefits for phobias and obsesssions when used alongside other treatments. It is also claimed to be useful in the treatment of narcolepsy, a condition in which people tend to fall asleep in quiet surroundings or whilst engaged in monotonous activities. It may take between two and four weeks before the symptoms of depression are relieved. During this time side effects may cause more problems and the feelings of depression may become worse.

Dosage Information

Adults (16 and over): Treatment begins with 10 mg daily, to be increased if necessary to **a maximum of 150 mg per day**. The usual maintenance dose is 30–150 mg daily in divided doses or as a single dose at bedtime.

Elderly and physically frail: The maximum recommended daily dose is 75 mg.

Children: Not recommended for the treatment of children.

OVERDOSE EXTREMELY DANGEROUS · SEEK IMMEDIATE MEDICAL HELP

Side Effects and Further Information
See pp. 70–73.

DESIPRAMINE

Trade name	Description
Pertofran	25 mg pale apricot-pink tablets marked EW.

General Information

Desipramine has similar effects and side effects to other tricyclic antidepressants but is said to be less likely to cause drowsiness. It may take between two and four weeks before the symptoms of depression are relieved. During this time the side effects are most likely to cause problems and the feelings of depression may be made worse.

Dosage Information

Adult (16 and over): Treatment begins with 75 mg daily in divided doses or as a single dose at bedtime, to be gradually increased if necessary to **a maximum dose of 200 mg**.

Elderly and physically frail: Initially 25 mg daily, to be gradually increased if necessary.

Children: Not recommended for children.

OVERDOSE EXTREMELY DANGEROUS · SEEK IMMEDIATE MEDICAL HELP

Side Effects and Further Information
See pp. 70–73.

DOTHIEPIN	
Trade name	*Description*
Prothiaden	25 mg red and brown capsules. 75 mg red tablets.

General Information

One of the antidepressants with more sedative properties, it can aid sleep or cause drowsiness. Like many of the antidepressants in this group it may take between two and four weeks to relieve the symptoms of depression.

Dosage Information

Adult (16 and over): Treatment begins with 75 mg in divided doses or preferably as a single dose at bedtime, to be increased if necessary to **a maximum dose of 150 mg per day**. Patients in hospital may receive up to 200 mg per day.

Elderly and physically frail: Treatment begins with 50–75 mg per day, to be increased, if necessary to **a maximum of 75 mg**.

Children: Not recommended for children.

OVERDOSE EXTREMELY DANGEROUS · SEEK IMMEDIATE
MEDICAL HELP

Side Effects and Further Information

See pp. 70–73.

DOXEPIN

Trade name	Description
Sinequan	10 mg orange capsules. 25 mg orange and blue capsules. 50 mg blue capsules. 75 mg yellow and blue capsules.

General Information

Doxepin has similar effects and side effects to other antidepressants but is more sedating. It can aid sleep or cause drowsiness. Doxepin is also prescribed for bedwetting in children. It may take between two and four weeks before the symptoms of depression are relieved.

Dosage Information

Adult (16 and over): Treatment begins with 75 mg per day in three divided doses. Doses of 100 mg or less per day may be taken as a single dose at bedtime. If necessary the dose may be increased gradually to **a maximum of 300 mg per day**.

Elderly and physically frail: Treatment begins with 10–50 mg per day and is increased gradually with caution. Many elderly people are likely to require no more than 30–50 mg per day.

Children: Not recommended for children under the age of 12.

> **OVERDOSE EXTREMELY DANGEROUS · SEEK IMMEDIATE MEDICAL HELP**

Side Effects and Further Information

See pp. 70–73.

IMIPRAMINE	
Trade name	*Description*
Tofranil	10 mg red-brown tablets. 25 mg red-brown triangular tablets. Syrup to be taken as directed by doctor or chemist.
Imipramine (generic name)	10 mg tablets. 25 mg tablets. Syrup to be taken as directed by doctor or chemist.

General Information

The first antidepressant manufactured and one of the more commonly prescribed, its effects and side effects are similar to other tricyclics but it is said to be less sedating. Imipramine is also prescribed for bedwetting in children. It takes between two and four weeks before any relief from symptoms is felt. During this time the side effects are most likely to be a problem and increase the feelings of depression.

Dosage Information

Adult (16 and over): Treatment begins with 75 mg per day in divided doses, to be increased gradually to **a maximum of 200 mg per day**. Hospital patients may receive higher doses. Daily doses of 150 mg or less may be taken as a single dose at bedtime.

Elderly and physically frail (60 and over): Treatment begins with 10 mg at night, increased if necessary with caution and close supervision to 10–25 mg three times a day. **The maximum dose is 75 mg per day**.

Children: Not recommended for the treatment of depression in children. Use in bedwetting only. This is a controversial approach to bedwetting. Imipramine only treats the physical side of the problem and parents and doctors should look to the psychological causes.

Dose of Imipramine Used in the Treatment of Bedwetting	
Age of child and body weight	Dose
6–7 years (20–25 kg/44–55 lbs)	25 mg before bedtime.
8–11 years (25–35 kg/55–77 lbs)	25–50 mg before bedtime.
Over 11 years (35–54 kg/77–119 lbs)	50–75 mg before bedtime.

The maximum dose is 75 mg, taken just before bedtime. Treatment should not exceed three months, *including* a period of gradual withdrawal from the drug. Bedwetting may resume when the drug is withdrawn, but treatment should not be resumed without a thorough physical examination of the child or in circumstances where other forms of help such as child guidance, counselling or psychological have not been attempted. The use of antidepressants as a treatment of bedwetting should ideally be regarded as a last resort.

> **OVERDOSE EXTREMELY DANGEROUS · SEEK IMMEDIATE MEDICAL HELP**

Side Effects and Further Information

See pp. 70–73.

IPRINDOLE	
Trade name	Description
Prondol	15 mg yellow tablets. 30 mg yellow tablets.

General Information

One of the less-often prescribed antidepressants whose effects and side effects are very similar to those of tricyclic antidepressants. It is said to cause less sedative effects. Particular caution is advised in prescribing this drug to people with liver disease. In rare circumstances iprindole may cause jaundice within the first 14 days of the drug being taken.

Dosage Information

Adult (16 and over): Treatment begins with 15–30 mg three times per day, to be gradually increased if necessary to **a maximum dose of 60 mg three times daily**. The usual maintenance dose is 30 mg three times per day.

Elderly and physically frail: Elderly and physically frail people should receive a lower initial dose.

Children: Not recommended for the treatment of children.

> **OVERDOSE EXTREMELY DANGEROUS · SEEK IMMEDIATE MEDICAL HELP**

Side Effects and Further Information

See pp. 70–73.

LOFEPRAMINE

Trade name	Description
Gamanil	75 mg round brownish-violet tablets.

General Information

One of the newer antidepressants and said to have milder side effects than older drugs. In comparison with other drugs in this group lofepramine does not appear to be substantially more effective. It takes between two and four weeks from the start of treatment before any relief from symptoms is felt. During this time the side effects are most likely to be a problem and increase the feelings of depression.

Dosage Information

Adult (16 and over): Between 140–210 mg per day in divided doses. The drug data sheet suggests that in severe cases of depression the doctor may prescribe higher doses on a try-it-and-see basis.

Elderly and physically frail: Lower doses are suggested for elderly people but these are not specified.

Children: The drug data sheet does not specify dose rates for children.

> OVERDOSE EXTREMELY DANGEROUS · SEEK IMMEDIATE
> MEDICAL HELP

Side Effects and Further Information

Said to be less severe than the older range of tricyclics. For further information, see pp. 70–73.

MAPROTILINE

Trade name	Description
Ludiomil	25 mg greyish-red tablets marked DP. 50 mg light orange tablets marked ER. 75 mg brownish-orange tablets marked ES.

General Information

A 'tetracyclic' antidepressant whose effects and side effects are broadly similar to those of tricyclic drugs. It is said that maprotiline may relieve the symptoms of depression more quickly than many of the antidepressants in this group, i.e. in two to three weeks. It can cause drowsiness and may help to induce sleep.

Dosage Information

Adult (16 and over): Treatment begins with 25–75 per day in three divided doses or as a single dose at bedtime. Increase if necessary with careful monitoring to **a maximum dose of 150 mg per day**.

Elderly and physically frail: Treatment begins with 10 mg three times per day or a single dose of 30 mg at bedtime. May be increased after one or two weeks to approximately half the normal adult dose.

Children: Not recommended for children.

> OVERDOSE EXTREMELY DANGEROUS · SEEK IMMEDIATE
> MEDICAL HELP

Side Effects and Further Information

Skin rashes are not uncommon and people have experienced fits after taking maprotiline. People with a history of epilepsy may be more likely to experience fits but this has also happened to people with no such history. For people suffering from mental disorders which include mania or feelings of persecution this drug may make these symptoms worse.

For further information see pp. 70–73.

MIANSERIN	
Trade name	*Description*
Bolvidon	10 mg white tablets marked CT4. 20 mg white tablets marked CT6. 30 mg white tablets marked CT7.
Norval	10 mg orange tablets marked 10. 20 mg orange tablets marked 20. 30 mg orange tablets marked 30.
Mianserin (generic name)	10 mg white tablets. 20 mg white tablets. 30 mg white tablets.

General Information

The effects and side effects are similar to those of older tricyclic antidepressants. The side effects of mianserin are said to be milder and less common. It exerts a sedative effect which may cause drowsiness or help to induce sleep. For the first three months of treatment the patient's blood should be tested every four weeks for signs of blood or liver disorders. If the patient develops a fever, sore throat or mouth infection whilst taking Mianserin the doctor should be notified immediately as this *may* be a symptom of a potentially dangerous drug reaction.

Dosage Information

Adult (16 years and over): Treatment begins with 30–40 mg per day in divided doses or as a single dose at bedtime, increased if necessary to **a maximum dose of 90 mg per day**. The usual maintenance dose is 30–90 mg per day.

Elderly and physically frail: Treatment begins with up to 30 mg per day, to be increased if necessary under close medical supervision. Elderly people are often treated with lower than usual doses.

Children: Not recommended for children.

> **OVERDOSE EXTREMELY DANGEROUS · SEEK IMMEDIATE MEDICAL HELP**

Side Effects and Further Information

Mianserin is said to have fewer and less frequent side effects than tricyclic antidepressants in general. It is, however, associated with more blood disorders than other drugs and can cause painful swellings in the joints of fingers and toes for a small number of people.

For further information see pp. 70–73.

NORTRIPTYLINE

Trade name	Description
Allegron	10 mg white tablets marked DISTA. 25 mg orange tablets marked DISTA.
Aventyl	10 mg yellow and white capsules marked H17. 25 mg yellow and white capsules marked H19. Liquid to be taken as directed by doctor or chemist.

General Information

A tricyclic antidepressant with similar effects and side effects to others in the group but said to be less sedating. It takes between two and four weeks from the start of treatment before any relief from symptoms is felt. During this time the side effects are most likely to be a problem and increase the feelings of depression.

Dosage Information

Adult (16 and over): Treatment begins with 20–40 mg per day in divided doses or as a single dose at bedtime. Gradually increase if necessary to **a maximum dose of 100 mg per day**. The usual maintenance dose is 30–75 mg per day.

Elderly and physically frail: Treatment begins with 30 mg per day and should be increased with great caution. Elderly people may respond to half the normal adult dose, and may experience side effects more severely.

Children: Not recommended for children as a treatment for depression. Adolescents may be treated for depression with a dose of between 30–50 mg per day in divided doses. Nortriptyline is sometimes used for the treatment of bedwetting.

Dose of Nortriptyline Used in the Treatment of Bedwetting	
Age of child and body weight	*Daily dose*
6–7 years (20–25 kg/44–55 lbs)	10 mg.
8–11 years (25–35 kg/55–77 lbs)	10–20 mg
Over 11 years (35–54 kg/77–119 lbs)	25–35 mg

The dose appropriate for the age and body weight of the child should not be exceeded. Treatment should not exceed a period of three months, including a period of gradual withdrawal from the drug. Bedwetting may return when the drug is withdrawn, but treatment with antidepressants should not be resumed without a thorough physical examination of the child or in circumstances where other forms of help such as child guidance have not been attempted.

> **OVERDOSE EXTREMELY DANGEROUS** · **SEEK IMMEDIATE MEDICAL HELP**

Side Effects and Further Information

Please note that nortriptyline is said to be less sedating. For further information, see pp. 70–73.

PROTRIPTYLINE

Trade name	Description
Concordin	5 mg salmon-pink tablets marked MSD26. 10 mg white tablets marked MD47.

General Information

One of the many tricyclic antidepressants with similar names and similar effects and side effects. Protriptyline does not cause sedation or drowsiness; in fact, it may have the opposite effect and cause problems with sleep. It takes between two and four weeks from the beginning of treatment before any relief from symptoms is felt. During this time the side effects are most likely to be a problem and increase the feelings of depression.

Dosage Information

Adult (16 and over): Treatment begins with 10 mg three to four times a day, increased if necessary to 60 mg. Once relief from depression is felt the dose should be gradually reduced. If the patient has sleeping difficulties it is recommended that the last dose should be taken before 4 pm. The usual maintenance dose is 15–60 mg per day.

Elderly and physically frail: Treatment begins with 5 mg three times a day, and should be increased with caution and close monitoring of the patient's condition. Doses higher than 20 mg per day increase the risk of the drug causing heart disorders.

Children: Protriptyline is not recommended for children under the age of 16.

> **OVERDOSE EXTREMELY DANGEROUS · SEEK IMMEDIATE MEDICAL HELP**

Side Effects and Further Information

Some side effects are more common with protriptyline than with other drugs in this group. These include increased anxiety; agitation; increased heart rate; reduced blood pressure; and increased photosensitivity, resulting in skin rashes after exposure to sunlight. Elderly people are more at risk of experiencing side effects, and of particular concern is the risk of heart damage.

For further information see pp. 70–73.

TRAZADONE

Trade name	Description
Molipaxin	50 mg violet and green capsules marked R365B. 100 mg violet and fawn capsules marked R365C. 150 mg pink tablets marked Molipaxin 150. Clear orange-flavoured liquid to be taken as directed by doctor or chemist.

General Information

Trazadone is not chemically related to the tricyclic antidepressants and appears to have some advantages over many of the drugs in this group. It can relieve the symptoms of depression within one week of beginning the treatment. Trazadone is also said to have fewer and less troublesome side effects. It has strong sedative effects which can cause drowsiness or promote sleep. Alcohol and tranquillizers taken at the same time as trazadone increase the sedative effect.

Dosage Information

Adult (16 and over): Treatment begins with 150 mg per day in divided doses after food or as a single dose at bedtime, increased if necessary to **a maximum dose of 300 mg per day**. Patients in hospital may be treated with up to 600 mg per day.

Elderly and physically frail: Treatment begins with 100 mg per day in divided doses after food or as a single dose at bedtime. Increase under supervision to 300 mg per day.

Children: Not recommended for children.

OVERDOSE EXTREMELY DANGEROUS · SEEK IMMEDIATE MEDICAL HELP

Side Effects and Further Information

Although Trazadone has fewer and less troublesome side effects than other antidepressants, it has on rare occasions caused priapism, a condition in which the penis becomes erect, possibly requiring surgery to return it to normal.

For further information see pp. 70–73.

TRIMIPRAMINE	
Trade name	*Description*
Surmontil	10 mg white tablets indented with Surmontil 10. 25 mg white tablets indented with Surmontil 25. 50 mg white and green capsules marked M&BSU50.

General Information

Surmontil is similar in its effects and side effects to other tricyclic antidepressants. It has a marked sedative effect which can induce slight drowsiness and promote sleep. It is said that Trimipramine can relieve the symptoms of depression within seven to ten days. Side effects are usually more pronounced at the beginning of treatment and until the drug has begun to reduce the feelings of depression there is a possibility that the depression may become more pronounced.

Dosage Information

Adult (16 and over): 50–75 mg per day taken as a single dose two hours before bedtime, *or* 25 mg at midday and 50 mg in the evening. Increase if necessary to **a maximum dose of 300 mg per day**. The usual maintenance dose is 75–150 mg per day.

Elderly and physically frail: Treatment begins with 10–25 mg three times per day. It is said that elderly people may benefit with a maintenance dose of half the normal adult dose.

Children: Trimipramine is not recommended for the treatment of children.

OVERDOSE EXTREMELY DANGEROUS · SEEK IMMEDIATE MEDICAL HELP

Side Effects and Further Information

See pp. 70–73.

VILOXAZINE	
Trade name	*Description*
Vivalan	50 mg white tablets marked v.

General Information

Once advertised by its manufacturers as 'the workers' antidepressant', Viloxazine is one of the newer antidepressants, said to relieve the symptoms of depression more quickly than many tricyclic antidepressants, and to have fewer and less severe side effects. It does not have a sedative effect; in fact if taken too late in the day it may cause patients difficulty in getting to sleep.

Dosage Information

Adult (14 and over): Treatment begins with 300 mg per day, taken 200 mg in the morning and 100 mg at lunchtime. The usual dose is 300 mg per day, **the maximum 400 mg per day**. The last dose of the day should not be taken after 6 pm.

Elderly: Treatment begins with 100 mg per day, to be increased if necessary under close supervision to normally half the adult dose.

Children: Not recommended for children under the age of 14.

> **OVERDOSE EXTREMELY DANGEROUS · SEEK IMMEDIATE MEDICAL HELP**

Side Effects and Further Information

Caution is required for people who suffer from epilepsy, particularly those taking phenytoin. Jaundice and convulsions have been reported in a small number of people.

For further information see pp. 70–73.

Tricyclic and Related Compounds: Side Effects and Further Information

Common Side Effects

Dry mouth. Tiredness. Blurred vision. Constipation. Nausea. Difficulty in urinating. Weight gain. *Not everyone finds these effects troublesome.*

Other Common Side Effects

Changes in heart rhythm. Reduced blood pressure leading to feelings of light-headedness, sweating, trembling and occasionally fainting. Reduced sexual feelings and difficulty in reaching orgasm. Men may also have difficulty in achieving or sustaining an erection. Less commonly some people become alarmingly excited and confused; these problems are more common in elderly people and children. *Not everyone experiences all or any of these effects.*

Less Common Side Effects

Black tongue. Obstruction of lower intestine. Epileptic fits. Agranulocytosis, a potentially fatal blood disorder. Leucopenia, a dangerous reduction of white blood cells. Eosinophilia, a blood disorder whose symptoms may include skin rashes and infections. Purpura and thrombocytopenia, which cause purple marks on the skin resembling bruising. Jaundice. *Very few people experience these effects.*

Overdose Symptoms

Confusion. Visual hallucinations. Dilated pupils. Reduction in body temperature. Hyperactivity. Seizure. Stiffening muscles. Coma. Heart failure.

OVERDOSE EXTREMELY DANGEROUS · SEEK IMMEDIATE MEDICAL ATTENTION

Withdrawal

Withdrawal from antidepressants should be done over a period of at least four weeks by a gradual reduction of the dose taken. If the drug has been taken for eight weeks or more, under no circumstances should the drug be stopped abruptly. Tricyclic antidepressants are not addictive but many people will experience withdrawal effects when they stop taking them. Withdrawing gradually from the drug gradually will prevent or minimize withdrawal effects.

Withdrawal effects: Nausea. Vomiting. Loss of appetite. Headache. Giddiness. Chills. Less commonly, extreme excitability, insomnia, panic, anxiety and restlessness have been reported.

How Tricyclic Antidepressants Interact with Other Drugs and Medicines

Tricyclic antidepressants interact with a wide range of other drugs. Be certain that your doctor, dentist or anaesthetist or anyone else who may prescribe or recommend medication for you is aware that you are taking an antidepressant.

DRUG	Result of interaction
Alcohol	Alcohol enhances the sedative effects of antidepressants, causing drowsiness.
Other antidepressants	MAOI antidepressants increase excitability and blood pressure, with potentially dangerous consequences. Fluoxetine increases the level of tricyclic antidepressant compounds in the blood.
Anti-epileptics, including barbiturates	The effectiveness of anti-epileptic drugs is reduced and the anti-epileptic drugs themselves reduce the effectiveness of tricyclic antidepressants.
Drugs to reduce blood pressure	The effectiveness of most drugs which reduce blood pressure is enhanced, but in *Ismelin, *Bethanidine, *Bendogen, *Esbatal, *Declinax and clonidine the effectiveness is reduced. There is an increased risk of high blood pressure if clonidine is withdrawn whilst the patient is taking a tricyclic antidepressant.

continued

Antihistimines (commonly found in over-the-counter cold remedies)	Increased sedation which may cause drowsiness.
Antipsychotic drugs (also known as major tranquillizers)	Increased side effects of both drugs (see pp. 157–162), in particular of drugs in the phenothiazine group, such as *Largactil.
Tranquillizers and sleeping pills such as *Valium, *Ativan, *Mogodon, etc	Increased side effects, in particular sedation or drowsiness.
Contraceptive pill and other sex-hormone-based drugs	Sex hormone drugs decrease the positive effects of antidepressants and increase their unpleasant side effects.
Disulfiram. *Antabuse, a drug used in the treatment of alcoholism	Increased level of the tricyclic antidepressant in the bloodstream. A potentially dangerous reaction to alcohol may arise if a patient is taking a tricyclic anti-depressant at the same time as Disulfiram.
Adrenaline, ephenedrine, isoprenaline, noradrenaline. Used in the treatment of heart disease	Potentially dangerous rises in blood pressure and changes in heart rate.
Cimetidine. *Tagamet, *Dyspamet, *Algitec. Used in the treatment of duodenal and gastric ulcers	Increased levels of antidepressant compounds in the blood stream.
Nitrates. Drugs used to treat angina and heart attacks, such as glyceryl trinitrate *Nitrocine, *Nitronal, *Tridil etc	Tricyclic antidpressants cause the mouth to dry, therefore reducing the effectiveness of drugs used to treat angina and heart attack by preventing them from being dissolved in the mouth as quickly.

*TRADE NAME

ALWAYS INFORM ANY NEW DOCTOR OR DENTIST WHO IS TREATING YOU THAT YOU ARE TAKING AN ANTIDEPRESSANT

Conditions in which Tricyclic Antidepressants Must be Avoided

Tricyclic antidepressants should not normally be prescribed to people who have had a recent heart attack, suffer from heart disease, are in an extremely excited state, or suffer from porphyria (a rare inherited blood disease).

Conditions in which Tricyclic Antidepressants Should be Used with Caution

Glaucoma (a condition in which there is high pressure inside the eye). Kidney disease. Epilepsy. Hyperthyroidism and when taking medicine for thyroid disease. Heart disease. Old age. Urination difficulties. They should also be used with caution for people expressing suicidal thoughts, and when receiving electo-convulsive therapy.

Use in Pregnancy

Tricyclic antidepressants should be avoided if possible during pregnancy, especially in the first or last three months, unless the depression is life-threatening. Extreme care is needed in balancing the needs of the mother against the risks to the unborn baby.

Use in Breast-feeding

Tricyclic antidepressants are carried from mother to baby in the breast milk, which can cause distress to the baby. Increased heart rates, irritability, muscle spasms and convulsions have been reported in newborn babies of mothers taking tricyclic antidepressants.

Dental Damage

Antidepressants inhibit the secretion of saliva and this causes tooth decay, mouth ulcers and changes in the tongue affecting the sense of taste. The dry mouth may persist after the drug has been stopped.

MAOI Antidepressants

Monoamine oxidase inhibitor (MAOI) antidepressants are a second-choice treatment for severely depressed people who fail to benefit from other treatments or treatment with tricyclic antidepressants. The name refers to the way they inhibit production of the enzyme which affects the production of 'monoamines', that is adrenaline, noradrenaline and serotinin, and others. The first MAOI antidepressant was iproniazid, which had previously been used as a treatment for tuberculosis. In the late 1940s it was noted that this drug caused elation in TB patients and this led to its being tried as an antidepressant. MAOI antidepressants have had a very chequered history, and a number of them, including iproniazid, have been withdrawn from use because they were discovered to be dangerous. They remain the focus of controversy with psychiatrists, as some believe they are useful whilst others believe that they have a very limited role, if any at all. Some patients treated with MAOIs become very agitated, occasionally losing contact with reality and becoming psychotic.

The major problem with these drugs is that if certain common foods, drinks and over-the-counter medicines are taken with them, the patient will experience a serious, and potentially but rarely fatal, reaction. The foods, drugs and drinks which must be avoided are listed on p. 84–87. It is extremely important that these dietary rules are kept to both whilst on MAOI antidepressants and for at least three weeks after they have been stopped. The dietary problems of these drugs are not, however, the sole reason for concern about their use. Withdrawal from MAOIs is more difficult than from tricyclics because the effects are likely to be more severe. The frequency of serious side effects is also higher with MAOIs. A study comparing the side effects of phenelzine (a MAOI), imipramine (a tricyclic) and a placebo (a dummy drug), showed that over a period of 33 weeks, 14 per cent of patients treated with the placebo reported a serious side effect, compared with 27 per cent of those on imipramine and 90 per cent of those on phenelzine. Of those treated with phenelzine, 10 per cent experienced a psychotic or near-psychotic episode, 8 per cent experienced a critical rise in blood pressure, 8 per cent had an increase in weight of over 15 pounds, and 22 per cent experienced impotence or the inability to reach orgasm. In all, 132 serious side effects were noted for 141 patients treated with phenelzine. The MAOIs are extremely dangerous in overdose, which, together with their serious side effects and hazards, means that they should never be prescribed as a drug of first resort to treat depression.

ISOCARBOXAZID

Trade name	Description
Marplan	10 mg pink tablets marked ROCHE.

FAST FACTS

Purpose	Treatment of depression
How do I take it?	30 mg daily as a single dose, or one 10 mg tablet three times per day. This may be increased under the close supervision of your doctor until the depression is relieved and later reduced gradually to the lowest dose which relieves the symptoms.
How long does it take to work?	Between one and four weeks.
Should I expect to experience side effects?	Yes, particularly when you first begin to take the drug. Not every one finds these side effects to be too troublesome, and many find them to become less so as time passes.
What are the most common side effects?	Dry mouth; drowsiness; nausea; headache; fatigue; restlessness; insomnia; constipation; blurred vision; swelling ankles.

continued

What should I do if I experience other distressing side effects?	Notify your doctor at once, particularly if you experience a sudden rise in temperature accompanied by a severe throbbing headache.
How long should I continue to take it?	This will depend on your needs and circumstances but you should review with your doctor your need to continue with the drug at least every six months. If the drug has not relieved your depression after six weeks you are unlikely to obtain any benefit from it.
Can I drive whilst taking it?	Antidepressants will affect your ability to drive safely.
Can I drink alcohol whilst taking it?	You should avoid red wines, lager and non-alcoholic beers. The drug will interact with any alcoholic drink and further impair your ability to drive.
Should I take any special precautions whilst taking it?	Yes, you must be careful to avoid certain foods, drinks, and medicines (see the list on p.84–87).
Is it addictive?	No, but you must withdraw from the drug gradually over a period of eight weeks or more in order to minimize the effects of withdrawal.

NEVER EXCEED THE PRESCRIBED DOSE · ALWAYS INFORM ANY DOCTOR, DENTIST OR ANAESTHETIST THAT YOU ARE TAKING A MAOI ANTIDEPRESSANT · BE CAREFUL ABOUT WHAT YOU EAT AND DRINK AND BE PARTICULARLY CAREFUL ABOUT ANY MEDICINES YOU BUY OR ARE PRESCRIBED · KEEP MEDICINES OUT OF THE REACH OF CHILDREN

General Information

Like other drugs in the MAOI group, isocarboxazid is most appropriately prescribed when no other antidepressant or chemical treatment has been effective. For a small number of people MAOIs sometimes bring rapid and pronounced relief from the symptoms of depression. For between 25 and 40 per cent of people they are unlikely to be of any benefit. Side effects are more common and more pronounced than with the tricyclic group of antidepressant drugs.

Dosage Information

Adult (16 and over): Treatment begins with 30 mg per day as a single dose or in three doses through the day. If the drug has not relieved the depression the dose may be gradually increased with great care and under close supervision to **a maximum dose of 60 mg per day for a period of no longer than six weeks**. If the depression has not been relieved after this time the drug should gradually be withdrawn as it will be unlikely to have any positive effect. At the higher dose levels there is a greater likelihood of serious side effects. Once the symptoms of the depression have been relieved the dose should gradually be reduced to the lowest level effective in relieving the depression.

Elderly and physically frail: It is recommended that elderly people should be treated at half the adult dose. Elderly people are more likely to suffer from side effects such as confusion, agitation and reduced blood pressure.

Children: Isocarboxazid is not recommended for children.

Side Effects and Further Information

Isocarboxazid, like the other MAOI antidepressants, is most definitely not the first-choice treatment amongst drug options for the treatment of depression. Its serious side effects and the way in which it interacts with other drugs and certain foods makes it a potentially hazardous treatment. It is said to be less likely to cause liver damage than phenelzine. For a fuller description of side effects, interactions with certain foods and other drugs, see pp. 84–87.

PHENELZINE

Trade name	Description
Nardil	15 mg orange tablets.

FAST FACTS

Purpose	Treatment of depression.
How do I take it?	One tablet three times daily, which may be increased to four tablets per day until the depression is relieved and later gradually reduced to as little as one tablet every other day.
How long does it take to work?	Between one and four weeks.
Should I expect to experience side effects?	Yes, particularly when you first begin to take the drug. Not every one finds these side effects to be too troublesome; and many people find them to become less so as time passes.
What are the most common side effects?	Dry mouth; drowsiness; nausea; headache; fatigue; restlessness; insomnia; constipation; blurred vision; swelling ankles.
What should I do if I experience other distressing side effects?	Notify your doctor at once, particularly if you experience a sudden rise in temperature accompanied by a severe throbbing headache.
How long should I continue to take it?	This will depend on your needs and circumstances but you should review with your doctor your need to continue with the drug at least every six months. If the drug has not relieved your depression after six weeks you are unlikely to obtain any benefit from it.
Is it addictive?	No, but you must withdraw from the drug gradually over a period of eight weeks or more in order to minimize its withdrawal effects.

continued

Can I drive whilst taking it?	Anitdepressants will affect your ability to drive safely.
Can I drink alcohol whilst taking it?	You should avoid red wines, lager and non-alcoholic beers. The drug will interact with any alcoholic drink and further impair your ability to drive.
Should I take any special precautions whilst taking it?	Yes, you must be careful to avoid certain foods, drinks, and medicines (see the list on pp. 84–87).

NEVER EXCEED THE PRESCRIBED DOSE · ALWAYS INFORM ANY DOCTOR, DENTIST OR ANAESTHETIST THAT YOU ARE TAKING A MAOI ANTIDEPRESSANT · BE CAREFUL ABOUT ANY MEDICINES YOU BUY OR ARE PRESCRIBED · KEEP MEDICINES OUT OF THE REACH OF CHILDREN

General Information

Phenelzine, like the other antidepressants of the MAOI type, is normally only prescribed if no other drug treatment has been effective. The side effects of MAOIs are more severe than those of other antidepressants, and because of their interactions with foods, drinks and medicines containing Tyramine (see p. 84–87), they are more hazardous. It can take up to four weeks before Phenelzine begins to relieve the symptoms of depression.

Dosage Information

Adult (16 and over): Treatment begins with one 15 mg tablet taken three times per day. An improvement *may* be experienced within one week. If there is no relief in the depression after a week the dose may be increased to **a maximum dose of one 15 mg tablet four times per day** (a total dose of 60 mg per day). People in hospital may be treated with a higher dose of up to two 15 mg tablets three times per day.

Elderly and physically frail: Same doses as above.

Children: Not recommended for children.

OVERDOSE EXTREMELY DANGEROUS · SEEK IMMEDIATE MEDICAL HELP

Side Effects and Further Information

A respected study has shown that over 90 per cent of patients treated with phenelzine over a period of 33 weeks had experienced at least one serious side effect. Thirty-eight per cent of patients experienced two or more serious side effects. Another study reported that the withdrawal effects of MAOIs are more severe than those of the tricyclic antidepressants. There is said to be a greater risk of a rare side effect of potentially fatal liver disease being caused by phenelzine than by other drugs in this group.

For further information on side effects, interactions with other drugs and foods, and cautions, see pp. 84–87.

TRANYLCYPROMINE

Trade name	Description
Parnate	10 mg Geranium red tablets marked SKF.

FAST FACTS

Purpose	Treatment of depression.
How do I take it?	10 mg twice daily in two doses the second dose must be taken no later than 3 p.m. This may be increased under the close supervision of your doctor until the depression is relieved and later reduced gradually to the lowest dose which relieves the symptoms.
How long does it take to work?	Between one and four weeks.
Should I expect to experience side effects?	Yes, particularly when you first begin to take the drug. Many people find that these side effects become less troublesome as time passes. Not every one finds these side effects to be too troublesome.

continued

What are the most common side effects?	Dry mouth; drowsiness; nausea; headache; fatigue; restlessness; insomnia; constipation; blurred vision; swelling ankles.
What should I do if I experience other distressing side effects?	Notify your doctor at once, particularly if you experience a sudden rise in temperature accompanied by a severe throbbing headache.
How long should I continue to take it?	This will depend on your needs and circumstances but you should review with your doctor your need to continue with the drug at least every six months. If the drug has not relieved your depression after six weeks you are unlikely to obtain any benefit from it.
Can I drive whilst taking the drug?	Antidepressants will affect your ability to drive safely.
Can I drink alcohol whilst I am taking the drug?	You should avoid red wines, lager and non alcoholic beers. The drug will interact with any alcoholic drink and further impair your ability to drive.
Should I take any special precautions whilst taking the drug?	YES YOU MUST BE CAREFUL TO AVOID CERTAIN FOODS, DRINKS, AND MEDICINES. See the list on pp.84–87.
Is it addictive?	POSSIBLY, it has a stimulant effect. You must withdraw from the drug over gradually over a period of eight weeks or more to minimise its withdrawal effects.

NEVER EXCEED THE DOSE YOUR DOCTOR PRESCRIBES · ALWAYS INFORM ANY DOCTOR, DENTIST OR ANAESTHETIST THAT YOU ARE TAKING A MAOI ANTIDEPRESSANT · BE CAREFUL ABOUT WHAT YOU EAT AND DRINK AND BE PARTICULARLY CAREFUL ABOUT ANY MEDICINES YOU BUY OR ARE PRESCRIBED · KEEP MEDICINES OUT OF THE REACH OF CHILDREN

General information

Tranylcypromine is described in the British National Formulary as "the most hazardous of the MAOIs because of its stimulant action." This stimulant effect has three potential dangers; some patients may become dangerously excited when they take the drug; some patients may become dependent on the drug because it makes them feel "high"; there is also a risk that patients might abuse the drug and expose themselves to the risk of fatal poisoning. If the treatment is effective it may take up to 3 weeks before the symptoms of the depression are relieved and another 1 or 2 weeks before the maximum benefit is obtained.

Dosage information

Adult (Age 16 and over): Treatment begins with 10 mg. taken twice daily not later than 3 p.m., increased after one week if necessary by raising the second dose of the day to 20 mg. Usual maximum dose per day 30 mg. Usual maintenance dose 10 mg per day.

Elderly and physically frail: Used with extreme caution in normal adult doses.

Side effects and further information

Tranylcypromine like the other MAOI antidepressants is most definitely not a treatment of first choice amongst the drug options for the treatment of depression. Its serious side effects and its interactions with other drugs and certain foods makes it a potentially hazardous treatment. Tranycypromine is said to be less likely to cause liver damage than phenelzine or isocarboxazid but more likely to cause a dangerous rise in blood pressure. For a fuller description of side effects, interactions with certain foods and other drugs see pages 84–87.

MAOI Antidepressants: Side Effects and Further Information

Common Side Effects

Dizziness. Reduced blood pressure. Blurred vision. Dry mouth. Feelings of weakness. Drowsiness. Constipation. Nausea. Vomiting. Insomnia. Oedema (a retention of bodily fluids which can cause swelling in the legs and ankles). Increased appetite and possibly a craving for sweet foods. Weight gain.

Less Common Side Effects

Headache. Sweating. Convulsions. Feelings of excitement. Neuritis (inflammation of the nerves). Difficulty with urination. Changes in behaviour. Reduced sexual feelings (in men impotence and difficulty in ejaculation). Changes in heart rhythm. Rashes. Trembling hands. Blood disease. Purpura (bruise-like blotches on the skin caused by the rupture of capillaries). Nervousness. Liver damage. Elderly people are more likely to experience these side effects and to experience them more severely.

Overdose Symptoms

Mania. Agitation. Coma. Reduced blood pressure or rapidly increased blood pressure. Bleeding into the brain.

> **OVERDOSE EXTREMELY DANGEROUS · SEEK MEDICAL ATTENTION**

Withdrawal

With the possible exception of tranylcypromine (Parnate), MAOI antidepressants are *not* addictive, but they must be withdrawn over a period of not less than four weeks in a gradual reduction of the dose. If the drug has been taken for a period of eight weeks or more, under no circumstances should it be stopped abruptly. A gradual withdrawal will prevent or minimize any withdrawal effects.

Withdrawal effects: Nausea. Vomiting. Loss of appetite. Giddiness. Insomnia. Feeling cold. Some people may become extremely agitated and prone to severe panic attacks or mania.

Important Dietary Precautions

The following is a list of foods, drinks and patent medicines which *must be avoided* whilst taking MAOI antidepressants:

Cheese, broad bean pods, pickled herrings, yoghurt, bananas, caviare, game (for example, hung pheasant, jugged hare, etc.) Bovril, Marmite, and any similar meat or yeast extracts.

Avoid red wines, in particular chianti, sherry and port. Be cautious of all beers, particularly lagers and non-alcoholic beers; some may be hazardous.

Avoid patent medicines sold in chemists and other shops. In particular avoid over-the-counter medicines for common colds and pain relief such as Nightnurse, Contact 400, Lemsip, Beecham's powders, etc. (Even if you are not taking a MAOI antidepressant these products may only be of marginal value to you. All have their own side effects.)

Always check with your doctor or pharmacist whether a drug is safe for you, whether it is prescribed for you or sold in a shop. This includes inhalants, suppositories, cough sweets, lozenges, nose drops and cough medicines. All of these may act as poisons to you if you use them whilst you are taking a MAOI antidepressant.

Symptoms of Reaction Between MAOI Drug and Certain Foods, Drinks and Medicines

Very severe throbbing headache, a rapid rise in blood pressure and a very high temperature.

SEEK URGENT MEDICAL ATTENTION

How MAOI Antidepressants Interact with Other Drugs and Medicines

DRUG	Result of Interaction
Pain killers such as codeine, diamorphine, diconal, dihydrocodeine, fortral, meptid, methadone, narphen, nubain, palfrium, pethidine, temgesic	Excitement or depression. Increased or decreased blood pressure.
Other MAOI antidepressants	An increase in the side effects and hazards associated with these drugs. (If a patient is to be changed from one MAOI antidepressant to another a period of at least ten days should pass between stopping one drug and starting another at a reduced dose.)
Tricyclic antidepressants	Excitability, increase in side effects and possibly an increased risk of potential hazards. Increased blood pressure. It is dangerous to take a MAOI antidepressant at the same time as, or within 14 days of, a tricyclic antidepressant. **The combination of tranylcypromine with clomipramine is very dangerous**.
Tryptophan	Excitability and confusion.
Drugs used to treat diabetes	The effect of Insulin and other antidiabetic drugs is enhanced.
Drugs used to treat blood pressure	Enhanced effects of drugs used to reduce blood pressure. With reserpine (*Decaserpyl, *Hypercal and *Serpasil), excitability and increased blood pressure.
Drugs used to treat epilspesy	MAOI antidepressants decrease the effectiveness of drugs prescribed to reduce convulsions. The manufacturers of carbamazapine (*Tegretol) recommend that the drug should not be taken with MAOI antidepressants or used within two weeks of taking a MAOI.

continued

Antimuscarinic drugs such as atropine, used to treat a variety of conditions including Parkinson's disease; Irritable bowel, and others.	Increased side effects.
Buspirone (trade name Buspar)	Increased blood pressure. It is recommended that buspirone should not be prescribed for people taking MAOI antidepressants.
Oxypertine (trade name Integrin). Used to treat serious mental distress such as schizophrenia	Excitability and a risk of a dangerous rise in blood pressure.
Levodopa (*Brocadopa and *Larodopa). Used in the treatment of Parkinson's disease	A serious risk of a dangerous rise in blood pressure.
Sympathomimetic drugs. Used in many treatments for the common cold. Also drugs like amphetamines, used *controversially* in the treatment of obesity and the control of hyperactive children	Risk of a dangerous increase in blood pressure.
Tetrabenazine (*Nitoman). Used to treat tics and other involuntary body movements caused by brain disorders	Excitability and a risk of a dangerous rise in blood pressure.

* TRADE NAME
ALWAYS INFORM ANY DOCTOR OR DENTIST TREATING OR PRESCRIBING FOR YOU THAT YOU ARE TAKING A MAOI ANTIDEPRESSANT.

Conditions in which MAOI Antidepressants Must be Avoided

Liver disease. Cerebrovascular diseases (disorders of the blood vessels and membranes of the brain). Phaeochromocytoma (a small tumour in the adrenal gland which causes attacks of raised blood pressure, increased heart rate palpitations and severe headaches). Porphyria (a rare inherited disorder causing skin inflammation or blistering under exposure to sunlight, stomach pains and mental disturbances). Tranylcypromine (*Parnate) should not be prescribed to people who suffer from hyperthyroidism.

Children, elderly and agitated people should *not* be treated with MAOI antidepressants.

Conditions in which MAOI Antidepressants Should be Used with Caution

Diabetes. Blood disease.

Use in Pregnancy and Breast-Feeding

MAOI antidepressants should be avoided in pregnancy and during breast-feeding unless the depression constitutes a severe risk to the mother or child and there is no other available form of treatment.

Compound Antidepressants

Although it is generally agreed that these drugs do not really have a place in the treatment of depression, some doctors believe that they should be tried for patients for whom no other treatment has proved effective. These compounds contain a mixture of two active drugs, an antidepressant and either an antipsychotic drug or a minor tranquillizer. According to the British National Formulary these compounds are *not* recommended because the doses of the ingredient drugs should be adjusted according to the needs of the individual patient. In the case of compound preparations which contain a minor tranquillizer with the antidepressant, there is a risk of addiction because although minor tranquillizers should not be taken for more than two weeks, drugs prescribed for depression are often taken over periods of months or even years. Compound antidepressants containing an antipsychotic drug also expose the patient to the long-term hazards of these drugs. Of particular concern here is the risk to the central nervous system, where damage can cause people to develop strange facial tics and other involuntary body movments (see the section on tardive dyskinesia, pp. 160–162). With both types of compound antidepressants the side effects associated with each constituent drug may be made worse by the way in which they interact. However, despite the fact that they are not recommended, compound antidepressants are available and are prescribed to a few people, as a treatment of last resort.

In the following list of compound antidepressants only a brief description of their effects and side effects is included. More information is available in the sections of the book describing the effects and side effects of major tranquillizers (pp. 157–162) and minor tranquillizers (pp. 28–29).

LIMBITROL

Trade name	Ingredients	Description
Limbitrol 5	12.5 mg amitriptyline (a tricyclic antidepressant); 5 mg chlordiazepoxide (a minor tranquillizer).	Pink and green capsules marked LOL5.
Limbitrol 10	25 mg amitriptyline; 10 mg chlordiazepoxide	Pink and dark green capsules marked LOL10.

FAST FACTS

Purpose	Treatment of depression.
Can I drink alcohol whilst taking it?	If you drink alcohol it will interact with the drug and further impair your ability to drive. It may make you feel ill.
How do I take it?	Capsules.
When do I take it?	Three tablets per day.
How long does it take to work?	Between two and four weeks.
Should I expect to experience side effects?	Yes. These may be more severe when you first begin to take the drug.
What are the most common side effects?	Dry mouth; drowsiness; less frequent urination; blurred vision; hangover; reduced sexual feelings.
What should I do if I experience other distressing side effects?	Notify your doctor.
How long should I continue to take it?	As this compound combines a minor tranquilizer, which would not normally be used for more than two weeks with an antidepressant which takes at least this time to work, it is impossible to say. You should discuss regularly your need to continue with this medication with your doctor.

continued

Is it addictive?	Yes, because it contains a minor tranquillizer. You should also be aware that you are likely to experience withdrawal symptoms when you stop taking any antidepressant. Withdrawal should be done gradually over a period of weeks.
Can I drive whilst taking it?	This compound will affect your ability to drive safely.

NEVER EXCEED THE PRESCRIBED DOSE · ALWAYS INFORM ANY DENTIST, DOCTOR OR ANAESTHETIST THAT YOU ARE TAKING THE DRUG · KEEP MEDICINES OUT OF THE REACH OF CHILDREN

Dosage Information

Adult (16 and over): Treatment begins with 5 mg three times per day, increased if necessary to 30 mg per day.

Elderly and physically frail: Not recommended.

Children: Not recommended for the treatment of children.

OVERDOSE EXTREMELY DANGEROUS · SEEK IMMEDIATE MEDICAL HELP

Side Effects and Further Information

As Limbitrol contains a minor tranquillizer and a tricyclic antidepressant, the side effects of both these groups of drugs may be experienced. For further information about side effects, see the section on minor tranquillizers (pp.28–29) and tricyclic antidepressants (pp. 70–73).

MOTIVAL

Trade name	Ingredients	Description
Motival	10 mg nortriptyline (a tricyclic antidepressant); 0.5 mg fluphenazine (a major tranquillizer)	Pink triangular tablets.

MOTIPRESS

Trade name	Ingredients	Description
Motipress	30 mg nortriptyline (a tricyclic antidepressant) 1.5 mg fluphenazine (a major tranquillizer)	Yellow triangular tablets.

FAST FACTS

Purpose	Treatment of depression
Is it addictive?	No, but you will experience withdrawal effects if you stop taking it suddenly. Withdrawal should be done gradually over a period of weeks.
How do I take it?	Tablets.
When do I take it?	Three times per day.
Should I expect to experience side effects?	Yes. These may be more severe when you first begin to take the drug.
What are the most common side effects?	Dry mouth; drowsiness; less frequent urination; blurred vision; hangover; reduced sexual feelings.
What should I do if I experience other distressing side effects?	Notify your doctor.
How long should I continue to take it?	This compound contains a major tranquillizer which when used over long periods of time carries a risk of causing a condition called tardive dyskinesia (see pp. 160–162). As the antidepressant it is combined with takes at least this time to work, it is impossible to say for how long the drug should be taken. You should discuss regularly your need to continue with this medication with your doctor.
Can I drink alcohol whilst taking it?	If you drink alcohol it will interact with the drug and further impair your ability to drive. It may make you feel ill.

continued

Can I drive whilst taking it?	This compound will affect your ability to drive safely.

NEVER EXCEED THE PRESCRIBED DOSE · ALWAYS INFORM ANY DENTIST, DOCTOR OR ANAESTHETIST THAT YOU ARE TAKING THE DRUG · KEEP MEDICINES OUT OF THE REACH OF CHILDREN

General Information

Motival and Motipress are compounds of identical ingredients mixed in different doses. As these products are not recommended by the British Medical Association or the Royal Pharmaceutical Society of Great Britain, they are presumably prescribed for depression which is resistant to any other form of treatment. The doses of the individual drugs which make up these compounds should be finely adjusted to meet the needs of the individual patient. Combining them in one tablet is a crude method of prescribing. Given the known side effects of the individual drugs and the known results of their interaction, the task of deciding whether the disadvantages of this medication outweigh its advantages is extremely difficult.

Dosage Information

Adult: Motival: One tablet three times daily. A total of three tablets per day.)

Motipress: one tablet at bedtime. (A total of one tablet per day.)

Elderly and physically frail: Motival: Treatment begins with one tablet twice daily. If no relief from symptoms is achieved at this dose, Motipress may be prescribed as an alternative in a dose of one tablet per day taken at bedtime.

Children: Not recommended for the treatment of children.

OVERDOSE EXTREMELY DANGEROUS · SEEK IMMEDIATE MEDICAL HELP

Side Effects and Further Information

As Motival and Motipress combine a tricyclic antidepressant with a major tranquilliser, the side effects of both these groups of drugs may be experienced. Apart from the known side effects and the results of interaction between the individual drugs, the potential risk of tardive dyskinesia must be considered. This may be a hazard more likely to effect elderly women, but tardive dyskinesia does occur in younger people of both sexes who take major tranquillizers over long periods. Tardive dyskinesia is described and discussed on pp. 160–162. The side effects of tricyclic antidepressants are described on pp. 70–73 and those of major tranquillizers on pp. 28–29.

PARSTELIN

Trade name	Ingredients	Description
Parstelin	10 mg tranylcypromine (a MAOI antidepressant); 1 mg trifluoperazine (a major tranquillizer)	Green tablets marked SKF.

FAST FACTS

Purpose	Treatment of depression.
How do I take it?	Tablets.
When do I take it?	Two or three tablets per day, taken one in the morning, one at midday and, if necessary, one at bedtime.
How long does it take to work?	Between one and four weeks.
Should I expect to experience side effects?	Yes. They may be more severe when you first begin to take the drug.
What are the most common side effects?	Dry mouth; drowsiness; less frequent urination; blurred vision; hangover; reduced sexual feelings.
What should I do if I experience other distressing side effects?	Notify your doctor.

continued

How long should I continue to take it?	This compound combines a major tranquillizer, which if used over long periods of time carries a risk of causing a condition called tardive dyskinesia (see pp. 160–162), with a MAOI antidepressant. You must avoid certain foods, drinks and drugs (see pp. 84–85). You should discuss regularly your need to continue with this medication with your doctor.
Is it addictive?	No, but you will experience withdrawal effects if you stop taking it suddenly. Withdrawal should be done gradually over a period of weeks.
Can I drive whilst taking it?	This compound will affect your ability to drive safely.
Can I drink alcohol whilst taking it?	Alcohol will further impair your ability to drive and may make you feel ill. You must be particularly careful of red wines, lager and non-alcoholic beers (see the section on MAOI antidepressants, pp. 84–85).

NEVER EXCEED THE PRESCRIBED DOSE · ALWAYS INFORM ANY DENTIST, DOCTOR OR ANAESTHETIST THAT YOU ARE TAKING THE DRUG · KEEP MEDICINES OUT OF THE REACH OF CHILDREN.

General Information

Parstelin combines a MAOI antidepressant with a major tranquillizer, drugs which should be prescribed separately at doses appropriate to the particular needs of the patient. Combining them in one tablet is a crude way of prescribing such powerful and potentially hazardous drugs. In the light of what is known about the side effects of these drugs and the way in which they interact, it is difficult to reach a decision as to whether any advantages of such medications outweigh their disadvantages. The manufacturers claim that these compound preparations bring faster relief from the symptoms of depression and anxiety than other antidepressants.

Dosage Information

Adult (16 and over): Treatment begins with two tablets per day, one taken in the morning and the other at midday. If this dose does not bring relief from symptoms a third tablet may be prescribed to reach **a maximum dose of three tablets per day**.

Elderly and physically frail: Extreme caution is needed in using Parstelin to treat elderly people. It should be avoided in patients with heart disease and epilepsy. There is an increased risk of tardive dyskinesia for elderly women. Tardive dyskinesia also occurs in young people who have been treated with major tranquillizers for long periods (for a fuller description of tardive dyskinesia and its side effects, see pp. 160–162).

Children: Not recommended for the treatment of children.

> **OVERDOSE EXTREMELY DANGEROUS · SEEK IMMEDIATE MEDICAL HELP**

Side Effects and Further Information

For more information about side effects, see the sections on MAOI antidepressants (pp. 83–85) and major tranquillizers (pp. 157–162).

TRIPTAFEN

Trade name	Ingredients	Description
Triptafen	25 mg amitriptyline (a tricyclic antidepressant); 2 mg perphenazine (a major tranquillizer)	Pink tablets marked AH/1D.
Triptafen M	10 mg amitriptyline (a tricyclic antidepressant); 2 mg perphenazine (a major tranquillizer)	Light pink tablets marked AH/2D.

FAST FACTS	
Purpose	Treatment of depression.
How do I take it?	Tablets.
When do I take it?	Three times per day.
How long does it take to work?	Between two and four weeks.
Should I expect to experience side effects?	Yes. These may be more severe when you first begin to take the drug.
What are the most common side effects?	Dry mouth; drowsiness; less frequent urination; blurred vision; reduced sexual feelings; feeling faint.
What should I do if I experience other distressing side effects?	Notify your doctor.
How long should I continue to take it?	This compound contains a major tranquillizer which if used over long periods of time carries a risk of causing tardive dyskinesia (see pp. 160–162). As the antidepressant it is combined with takes at least this long to work, it is impossible to say for how long the drug should be taken. You should discuss regularly your need to continue with this medication with your doctor.
Is it addictive?	No, but you will experience withdrawal effects if you stop taking it suddenly. Withdrawal should be done gradually over a period of weeks.
Can I drive whilst taking it?	This compound will affect your ability to drive safely.
Can I drink alcohol whilst taking it?	It will further impair your ability to drive and may make you feel ill.

NEVER EXCEED THE PRESCRIBED DOSE · ALWAYS INFORM ANY DENTIST, DOCTOR OR ANAESTHETIST THAT YOU ARE TAKING THE DRUG · KEEP MEDICINES OUT OF THE REACH OF CHILDREN.

General Information

Triptafen is a combination of a tricyclic antidepressant and a low-dose major tranquillizer. The British National Formulary emphasises that the use of compound antidepressants like Triptafen is *not* recommended. Because the constituent drugs in these compounds have their own side effects, and each interacts with the other, they should be prescribed separately in doses carefully matched to the needs of the individual. These products represent a form of bulk prescribing, based on the assessed needs of a defined group of patients and the size of the market for the product. Another way of seeing them is as 'off the peg' prescriptions. Most of us buy 'off-the-peg' clothes and are very satisfied with them; if they don't fit too well we can always take them in or let them out a bit for comfort or vanity. With 'off-the-peg' prescriptions, however, it is simply not possible to make minor alterations to the effects and side effects of the drugs. These compound drugs have maintained a small but secure niche in the marketplace for some years; and it is safe to assume that they satisfy the clinical requirements of the doctors who prescribe them as well as the clinical needs of their patients. According to the manufacturers, Triptafen is most appropriately prescribed to people who suffer mild to moderate depression, accompanied by anxiety.

Dosage Information

Adult (16 and over): Triptafen: one tablet taken three times per day. If necessary a fourth tablet can be added to the daily dose, usually taken at bedtime. If the drug has not relieved the symptoms of depression within four weeks it is time to consider an alternative form of treatment.

Triptafen M: As above.

Elderly and physically frail: As with other antidepressants, extra caution is required in prescribing these drugs to elderly people. Elderly women may be more vulnerable than others to the risk of tardive dyskinesia developing after periods of treatment with major tranquillizers (For a fuller description of tardive dyskinesia and its side effects, see pp. 160–162).

Children: Not recommended for the treatment of children aged 14 or younger.

OVERDOSE EXTREMELY DANGEROUS · SEEK IMMEDIATE
MEDICAL ATTENTION

Side Effects and Further Information

For further details of the side effects of both ingredients in this compound, see the section on pp. 70–73 and major tranquillizers (pp. 157–162).

Other Drugs Used in the Treatment of Depression

FLUOXETINE	
Trade name	*Description*
Prosac	20 mg white and off green capsules marked 3105.

General Information

Fluoxetine is a relatively new antidepressant and is not chemically related to any of the older antidepressants. Unlike many other antidepressants, it does not cause drowsiness or sedation; in fact it appears to have an alerting effect, also causing nervousness, tremors and insomnia. Its launch on the market was accompanied by the usual chorus of claims of its superiority over existing drugs, and almost as predictably it has more recently become the centre of a controversy over its safety. The concern over its safety is focused on a suspicion that it may make some patients suicidal. Six case studies were recently published in America of patients who became obsessively suicidal whist taking fluoxetine. These studies have been criticized by other doctors, who have pointed out amongst other things that in four of the cases the patients were also taking other psychiatric drugs. So far none of the drug-monitoring bodies such as the Committee on the Safety of Medicines have thought it necessary to take any action in this controversy. However, it is generally accepted that the adverse effects of drugs tend to be under-reported and that the monitoring of such effects is far from being sensitive.

There appears to be some confusion surrounding the use of fluoxetine. The British National Formulary recommends a dose of 20 mg per day, whilst the current Data Sheet Compendium contains the following unedifying advice to prescribers: 'A dose of 20 mg/day is recommended. Although Prosac has been administered at doses of up to 80 mg/day, available data show that most patients do not require more than 20 mg daily. The maximum daily dose should not exceed 80 mg.' In a recent Channel 4 TV documentary, a learned professor of psychopharmacology commenting on the Prosac controversy said: 'The jury remains out.' In the meantime, the uncertainty about the drug's safety remains, and whilst the drug's manufacturers recommend the use of one dose, they also suggest that a dose four times higher might be used. Thus, the average doctor or psychiatrist, who may or may not keep abreast of the scientific evidence about the nature, purposes, effects and use of drugs, is left in the majestic solitude of his or her clinical judgement, whilst the patient is left, as always, in the dark.

What can be said about fluoxetine is that it appears much less dangerous in overdose than other antidepressants and its side effects are different and apparently less severe. From a study published in 1987 which compared the progress of 28 patients on fluoxetine with 32 patients on imipramine, it appears that fluoxetine is as effective as imipramine in its capacity to relieve the symptoms of depression. Ten patients withdrew from the trial; five simply stopped attending (four were on fluoxetine, one on imipramine); three withdrew because they felt they were getting no benefit from the drugs (two were on fluoxetine, one on imipramine); and two stopped because they found the side effects intolerable (both were on fluoxetine). The fluoxetine group was more likely to be troubled by tremors, insomnia, weight loss and nausea, whilst the imipramine group was more likely to be troubled by weight gain, constipation, headaches and dry mouth. All these side effects were described as being 'minor' by the authors of the study.

Dosage Information

Adult (16 and over): 20 mg per day (see above under General Information).

Elderly and physically frail: The maximum dose should not exceed 60 mg per day.

Children: Not recommended for the treatment of children.

OVERDOSE EXTREMELY DANGEROUS · SEEK IMMEDIATE MEDICAL HELP

Side Effects and Further Information

Fluoxetine may cause a wide variety of side effects. If a rash develops it is recommended that the drug be stopped as this could be symptomatic of vasculitis (the inflammation of small blood vessels), anaphylaxis (an allergic reaction), inflammation of the lung or fibrosis (a scarring of tissues following injury or inflammation). Nausea. Vomiting. Diarrhoea. Loss of appetite, leading to weight loss. Headache. Nervousness. Insomnia. Anxiety. Tremors. Dry mouth. Dizziness. Hypomania (elated mood, uninhibited behaviour, rapid speech and abnormal energy). Drowsiness. Convulsions. Fever. Sexual difficulties. Sweating. Less common side effects are blood changes and reduced white blood cell count. Other side effects reported are: Vaginal bleeding after withdrawal of the drug. Anaemia. Thrombocytopenia (a blood disorder which may cause bleeding into the skin, leading to bruise marks and in the event of an injury a tendency to increased bleeding). Confusion.

Use with caution in patients with liver or kidney disease, epilepsy and diabetes. Avoid in pregnancy and in breast-feeding mothers.

It may impair driving ability.

FLUPENTHIXOL	
Trade name	*Description*
Fluanxol (see also Depixol, p. 125)	0.5 mg red tablets marked Lundbeck in black. 1 mg red tablets marked Lundbeck in white.

General Information

Fluanxol is a low-dose preparation of flupenthixol, which is more often used to treat conditions such as schizophrenia. The use of flupenthixol in depression is a short-term, last resort approach when all other treatments and drugs have failed. When used in low doses it is said that flupenthixol has few side effects compared with antidepressants, and it is not as dangerous in overdose. As it is used in the short-term treatment of depression at doses of approximately one-sixth of those used for schizophrenia, the side effects should be less frequent and less severe and the risk of tardive dyskinesia should be low. For fuller information about flupenthixol, see p. 125. Flupenthixol is not recommended for severe or agitated depression or mania. The drug is claimed to exert its antidepressant action within two to three days. If no relief of the depression has been obtained after one week the drug should be withdrawn. It may impair driving ability.

Dosage Information

Adult (16 and over): Treatment begins with 1 mg per day, given in one dose in the morning, which may be increased if necessary after one week to 2 mg per day. **The maximum dose for depression is 3 mg per day**. If doses of more than 2 mg per day are given, divided doses should be used, and the last dose should be given no later than 4 pm as the drug may impair sleep if taken later.

Elderly and physically frail: Treatment begins with 0.5 mg per day, given as a single dose in the morning, which may be increased if necessary to 1 mg per day. If any further increase in the dose is considered great care must be exercised. Although this is rare, **the maximum dose of 2 mg per day** may be given in divided doses of 1 mg in the morning and 1 mg at about 4 pm.

Children: Not recommended for children.

> **OVERDOSE EXTREMELY DANGEROUS · SEEK IMMEDIATE MEDICAL HELP**

Side Effects and Further Information

See the entry on flupenthixol, p. 125.

FLUVOXAMINE

Trade name	Description
Faverin	50 mg yellow tablets marked Duphar 291. 100 mg yellow tablets.

General Information

Fluvoxamine is another recently introduced antidepressant which was launched with the usual claims of superiority over existing drugs and has since run into controversy. At its launch, fluvoxamine was said by its manufacturers to be useful for a wide range of human problems accompanied by low moods, from aches, pains and worries to psychosomatic illnesses. In 1988, following the deaths of five patients taking fluvoxamine, the Department of Health issued a warning to doctors. At that time over 1,000 reports of adverse effects with fluvoxamine had been received by the Committee on the Safety of Medicines, ranging from nausea and vomiting to convulsions.

Fluvoxamine is now recommended to treat the symptoms of depressive illness. It should not be used by people with a history of epilepsy. It is less dangerous in overdose and it is said to have less serious and fewer side effects than older antidepressants.

Dosage Information

Adult (16 and over): 100–200 mg per day. 100 mg may be given as a single dose in the evening, but if a dose higher than 100 mg per day is given, it should be taken in divided doses. **The maximum dose is 300 mg per day**.

Elderly and physically frail: The elderly and physically frail should receive adult doses.

Children: Not recommended for the treatment of children.

OVERDOSE EXTREMELY DANGEROUS · SEEK IMMEDIATE MEDICAL HELP

Side Effects and Further Information

Fluvoxamine frequently causes nausea, vomiting and diarrhoea. Less frequently it may cause drowsiness, giddiness, agitation, anxiety, headaches and tremors. Bradycardia (the slowing of the heart beat to less than 50 beats per minute) and convulsions have also been reported. Fluvoxamine should be used with caution in pregnancy and breast-feeding and in patients with liver and kidney disease. It should not be taken by anyone with a history of epilepsy. It may impair driving ability.

TRYPTOPHAN

Trade name	Description
Optimax	500 mg yellow capsule-shaped tablets marked OPTIMAX and containing vitamins. Chocolate-flavoured powder to be mixed with warm milk or water.
Optimax WV	500 mg yellow capsule-shaped tablets marked OPTIMAX WV (without vitamins).
Pacitron	500 mg oblong yellow-orange tablets marked PCT500.

General Information

Tryptophan products have been withdrawn from use and are only available on a named patient basis for the treatment of serious depression where no other treatment or drugs are effective. Tryptophan was withdrawn from use following reports of its causing eosinophilia-myalgia (a blood condition in which certain white blood cells increase in number, with dangerous consequences). As a last-resort treatment tryptophan may be used for short periods of time, either alone or with a MAOI antidepressant. The use of tryptophan should be reviewed every three months.

Dosage Information

Adult (16 and over): 1–2 g per day after meals. When taken with a MAOI antidepressant, 500 mg per day for one week and gradually increased.

Elderly and physically frail: The elderly and physically frail should receive adult doses.

Children: Not recommended for the treatment of children.

> **OVERDOSE EXTREMELY DANGEROUS · SEEK IMMEDIATE MEDICAL HELP**

Side Effects and Further Information

Tryptophan should be used with caution in the following conditions: Bladder disease. Nutritional deficiency, in particular of pyridoxine (vitamin B_6). The dose should be lower when used with MAOI antidepressants and tryptophan should be withdrawn if the patient suffers from headaches or blurred vision.

Introduction

Antipsychotic drugs are used to control psychoses, that is symptoms such as hallucinations, delusions, irrational fixed ideas of persecution, and social withdrawal.

When a person experiences a florid psychotic state he or she is said to have lost contact with reality. Such symptoms occur in a wide variety of conditions including severe depression, manic depression and brain disorders caused by injury or disease. The most commonly diagnosed and best known psychotic condition in which these drugs are used is schizophrenia which is discussed below. The same compounds are also used in low doses to treat anxiety, nausea and vomiting. Antipsychotic drugs are amongst the most widely prescribed and important drugs in psychiatry.

They are commonly referred to as 'major tranquillizers', but the term 'tranquillizer' is misleading: antipsychotics can relieve the symptoms of serious mental illness but they do not induce tranquillity. In fact, very often they have quite the opposite effect of causing restlessness and agitation, making it difficult for people to stand or sit still. Antipsychotic drugs are also referred to as 'neuroleptics'. This term, which means a treatment that finely tunes the nerves, or state of mind, is also misleading: these drugs have a wide range of powerful physical and psychological effects which are not limited to the symptoms for which they are prescribed. The effects are not predictable for any given individual and they are not fully understood. In fact, the side effects of antipsychotic drugs are often severe enough to merit treatment with other drugs, and they in turn have their own troublesome side effects and problems. The terms 'tranquillizer' and 'neuroleptic' are misnomers and seriously understate the actual effects of the drugs on those who take them. For these reasons this guide uses the more neutral term 'antipsychotic' to describe them.

The first of the antipsychotics, chlorpromazine, was derived from a substance called phenothiazine which was discovered in 1883. Phenothiazine was used in the mid-1930s as an insecticide, a treatment for parasitic worms and as an antiseptic for the bladder. Chlorpromazine was first used in surgery to improve the effects of anaesthetics. In 1952 French researchers described how chlorpromazine produced an effect which they described as 'artificial hibernation.' They noted that whilst patients administered Chlorpromazine did not lose consciousness, they did have a tendency to become sleepy and showed a marked lack of interest in what was going on around them. The first trials of Chlorpromazine for psychiatry showed that it was effective in reducing the symptoms of schizophrenia and other types of mental agitation. As the first effective antipsychotic drug, chlorpromazine transformed the face of psychiatry.

Before the advent of chlorpromazine mental hospitals provided little more than restraint and a range of treatments which were often hazardous and rarely effective. A booklet produced for doctors by a leading manufacturer of antipsychotic drugs makes the following observation: 'People with experience in psychiatric care agree that the introduction of Chlorpromazine in psychiatric hospitals has reduced the time patients spend in seclusion and restraint.' However, other people with experience of psychiatric care argue that this change may be more cosmetic than real and that drugs like chlorpromazine can be used as an alternative and insidious method of seclusion and restraint. Antipsychotic drugs represent an important advance in improving the quality of life for many thousands of seriously distressed people, but their effectiveness is frequently overstated whilst their problems are too often overlooked.

It has been claimed that the introduction of chlorpromazine and its chemical cousins led directly to the reduction of the numbers of people confined in mental hospitals. However, a more careful reading of history shows that the decline in the number of psychiatric in-patients began soon after the end of World War II, some ten years before the introduction of Chlorpromazine. Antipsychotic drugs undoubtedly added impetus to the movement towards treatment in the community.

Chlorpromazine (trade name Largactil) remains one of the most widely prescribed of the antipsychotic drugs. Since it was first introduced many similar drugs have been put on the market by the pharmaceutical industry. There are those who believe that there are now far too many similar compounds available. They argue that rational prescribing is made difficult by the plethora of 'me too' drugs competing for the attention and loyalties of the doctors who will prescribe them. There are no significant differences in the antipsychotic properties of these drugs, although there are differences between the severity of some of their side effects. Thus the choice as to which drug should be prescribed to a particular patient will depend more on its side effects than on any other factor. Currently there are 36 antipsychotic products listed in the British National Formulary. Chlorpromazine as the first of the antipsychotic is the one against which the effects of the others are compared for reference.

Antipsychotic drugs may be taken by mouth in tablet form or as a syrup, or by injection. Depot antipsychotics such as Fluphenazine (Modecate) and Flupenthixol (Depixol) are administered by injection and their effects can last for several weeks. They may be administered at intervals of between one and four weeks, and people who need to observe religious dietary laws may wish to know that the active drug is suspended in sesame oil. The advantage of depot drugs is that the patient does not have to remember to take pills regularly, and in ideal circumstances, once the dose level of a depot antipsychotic has been established no other similar drug should be necessary. However, many patients regularly receive two or more antipsychotic drugs in the same course of treatment, which exposes them to an increased number of side effects and seldom brings any real advantage.

Antipsychotic drugs do not work for every one and neither do they always prevent people who take them regularly from suffering relapses. An English study (Leff and Wing, 1971)[1] which looked at a very large number of people diagnosed as schizophrenic revealed that seven in one hundred did not have any positive response to antipsychotic drugs and that twenty-four out of a hundred relapsed within a year of taking them. American research (Cole, Goldberg and Klerman, 1964) shows that one patient in twenty failed to show any positive response and that between one in ten and one in five relapsed whilst taking the medication within the first six months of treatment.[2] Recent research (Crow et al., 1986) which compared the progress of people who after their first episode of schizophrenia took a 'placebo' with those who took a real antipsychotic drug found that within two years 58 per cent of

[1]Less, J. P. and Wing, J. K.: 'Trial of Maintenance Therapy in Schizophrenia, *British Medical Journal*, 5, pp.559–604, 1971.

[2]Cole, J. O., Goldberg, S. C. and Klerman, G. L.: 'Phenothiazine Treatment in Acute Schizophrenia', *Archives of General Psychiatry*, 10, pp.246–61, 1964.

those taking the real drug had relapsed whilst 78 per cent of those receiving the placebo had relapsed.[3] Findings like these show that most patients are likely to benefit for most of the time from taking antipsychotic medication. But such findings do not support the enthusiasm with which these drugs are prescribed by many psychiatrists – often two or more at the same time and frequently in very high doses. Neither do such findings support the case of those who want to extend the legal powers of psychiatrists to treat people forcibly with these drugs in the community.

Antipsychotic drugs do not affect every patient in the same way; different people may require different doses to achieve a maximum control of symptoms with a minimum of side effects. This means that when a person is first prescribed a drug, the dose should begin as low as possible and be increased until the maximum control of symptoms has been achieved. In ideal circumstances the dose should then be reduced to the minimum that will maintain the maximum control of symptoms. Some people will require much higher doses than others and some will also experience much more severe side effects. Generally speaking, the higher the prescribed dose, the more likely it is that the side effects will be severe. Many patients are routinely prescribed very high doses of antipsychotic drugs, a practice which is difficult to understand given that research into the use of such doses shows that patients are unlikely to benefit from them. Patients treated with megadoses of antipsychotic drugs will at the very least be unnecessarily exposed to more severe side effects and an increased risk of neurological damage.

In a recent study into psychiatric prescribing practices (Johnson and Wright, 1990) the authors reviewed the research undertaken to establish whether very high doses of antipsychotics may be more effective, particularly to those patients who do not benefit from standard doses. They concluded that 'The consensus view is that very high doses have not proved beneficial.' In the same paper, they cited a number of reports which showed that very high doses of antipsychotic drugs actually made some patients' symptoms worse.[4] In the light of

[3]Crow, T. J., MacMillan, J. S., Johnson, A. L. and Johnson, E. C.: 'The Northwick Park Study of First Episodes of Schizophrenia; A Controlled Study of Neuroleptic Treatment'; British Journal of Psychiatry, 148, pp.120–7.

[4]Johnson, D. A. W., and Wright, N. F.: 'Drug Prescribing for Schizophrenic Out-Patients on Depot Injections: Repeat Surveys over 18 years', British Journal of Psychiatry, 156, pp.827–34, 1990.

a great deal of research which has failed to show any substantial benefits from using very high doses it is difficult to understand why so many psychiatrists continue to prescribe them in this way. It may be considered the only recourse for patients whose symptoms are not improved by the use of antipsychotic drugs within the normal dose range. There are also those who believe that high doses may be administered simply in order to sedate people and give the medical staff a quiet life. Whatever the reasons, it is a matter for grave concern. Antipsychotic drugs are sometimes referred by patients to as 'the chemical cosh' or 'the liquid strait-jacket'. This too is a matter for strong concern, not only because the use of such terms may point to the abuse of these drugs, but also because they may put off people who might benefit from them.

Under the provisions of the 1983 Mental Health Act drugs may be administered by force to protesting patients (for details of consent procedures under the MHA, 1983, see p.186-189). Quite often pressure may be exerted on people by nurses and others to make them take the drugs. There are circumstances in which it may be necessary for the safety and well-being of a mentally distressed person, or for the safety of others, that drugs should be administered without the patient's consent. These factors of compulsion and pressure create powerful moral obligations for those responsible for the administration of such drugs. There is an obligation to be as sure as possible that the benefits of the drug will substantially outweigh any disadvantages and risks to the patient. This demands an awareness and sensitivity to the patients' experiences of the drug's effects.

Organizations like MIND receive many enquiries and complaints from patients and relatives about distressing side effects, excessive doses and indifference amongst psychiatrists and nurses. To become a psychiatric patient often means becoming a non-citizen and being rendered invisible behind a diagnostic label. Once a person has been labeled a 'schizophrenic' it is often wrongly assumed that he or she is totally unable to make any rational choices or decisions. Any complaint that such a person makes about his or her treatment is likely to be perceived as being 'paranoid'. People who suffer from schizophrenia often do have paranoid ideas, but they are also vulnerable to poor or inadequate standards of treatment. It is well to remember that most of the reforms in psychiatric care have been generated by scandals involving the neglect or ill-treatment of psychiatric patients.

Getting the Most from Antipsychotic Drugs

This introduction has focused a great deal on the problems of these drugs and the way they are used both in psychiatric hospitals and in the community. This is inevitable and necessary. It is inevitable because there is not so much ground to cover in describing the useful effects of the drugs. It is necessary because people have a need and a right to adequate information about the drugs that are prescribed for them. There is a great deal of evidence which points to the best way to use antipsychotic drugs in order to achieve the best possible relief of symptoms and the least problems with side effects and long-term risks. It is necessary to do so because people need and have a right to adequate information about the drugs they themselves or those close to them are prescribed, and there is a great deal of evidence which points to the best way to use antipsychotic drugs in order to get the greatest possible relief of symptoms and the fewest possible side effects and long-term risks.

In conditions like schizophrenia it is usually necessary for the patient to continue taking antipsychotic drugs over long periods. For some people it may mean taking the drugs for the rest of their lives. When treatment begins it is usually best to start with the lowest dose which achieves the best possible relief of symptoms. It is recommended that the drug is started at the lowest end of its dosage range and gradually increased until the appropriate dose for the individual patient has been established. Many people will experience the common side effects of these drugs very early on in their treatment, and if these are troublesome another drug may be prescribed to counter them (for details of medications for side effects, see p.165). Some psychiatrists routinely prescribe medication for side effects at the same time as they prescribe an antipsychotic, but this is not wise. Medications for side effects can reduce the effectiveness of antipsychotic drugs and increase their long-term hazards. As a general rule, it is agreed not only that it is usually best to prescribe antipsychotic drugs at the lowest effective dose, but that this should be done with as few other drugs as possible. Once the symptoms have been controlled, it may be possible for the dose of the antipsychotic to be reduced without the symptoms getting worse.

Some patients forget to take their pills regularly and others may unwisely stop taking them, and there are also patients with schizophrenia who may develop a fixed belief that their doctors or families are poisoning them with the drugs (although such a belief is not in itself sufficient reason to resort to enforcing treatment). For these reasons patients receiving antipsychotic medication may be given 'depot' injections which last for weeks at a time. These patients may receive their injections in their own homes from a community psychiatric nurse, or they may attend a monthly special clinic to receive their injections. Many patients in hospitals also receive their antipsychotic drugs by monthly injection. There is no advantage to the patient in combining depot with other antipsychotic compounds, as when prescribed in this way the range and severity of side effects are likely to be increased.

Antipsychotic drugs may also be used in emergencies when people are very disturbed. Even whilst on the drugs some patients may, as a result of stress, become agitated and disturbed, and in these circumstances an extra injection of another antipsychotic drug can be given to deal with the crisis. The injection may not be aimed simply at the psychiatric symptoms but also at the behaviour of the patient. The drug will reduce the problem behaviour, and it will also have the effect of bringing the patient to a state of manageable lethargy. Whilst this is far from being an ideal solution, it is sometimes the only means available to deal with a potential crisis.

Many patients are prescribed antidepressants with antipsychotic drugs. Some antipsychotic drugs can cause patients to feel depressed and some people who suffer from schizophrenia may feel depressed. However, the combination of antipsychotic and antidepressant medications is controversial. In reviewing the studies of such combination prescribing, Johnson and Wright (1990) conclude, 'It is clear that at present time the prescription of antidepressants must be regarded as a therapeutic trial. Since there are possible risks of schizophrenic deterioration these patients must receive careful supervision.'[5]

There is a growing amount of evidence that antipsychotic drugs are a great deal more effective when given as part of a comprehensive treatment plan which includes help with the daily problems of living. Stress is a major factor in causing people who suffer from schizophrenia to relapse. An inevitable consequence of serious mental illness is that it causes a great deal of anguish and stress to those closest to the sufferer. If all these stresses are not dealt with the chances of the patient experiencing a serious relapse are considerably increased. The families of mentally ill people often need help and understand-

---

[5]Johnson, D. A. W. and Wright, N. F.: op. cit., p. 830.

ing in order to cope with the strains imposed on them and when this help is given it can be extremely effective in preventing relapses.

There is an increasing number of studies which show that the relapse rate amongst patients who receive social support as well as drugs is dramatically less than amongst those who receive drugs only. Two recent studies are worthy of mention. In the first (Leff et al, 1982, and also referred to in 1989 study by Falloon et al)[6] the progress of two groups of people diagnosed as schizophrenic was monitored over two years. One group received antipsychotic drugs only, whilst the other received antipsychotic drugs at the same time as their families were given help with dealing with their emotional problems. After two years more than three-quarters of those who received only the drug had suffered a serious relapse, whilst only one-fifth of those who had received the drug and family suppport had relapsed over the same period. The second study, compared the relapse rates of two similar groups of patients also over a two-year period. This time, 83 per cent of those on drugs only had relapsed, compared to 17 per cent of those who had received drugs and family support. Few hospitals or community teams seem to have the skills and resources to provide this sort of service. For most people the drugs-only regime is all that is available. It is to be hoped that knowledge of such encouraging findings will stimulate people who suffer from mental illness to work with their relatives and, in turn, to make demands for more comprehensive services. Apart from preventing unnecessary distress to patients and their relatives, approaches such as those outlined above may save money by reducing the need for people to be admitted to hospital.

[6]Leff, J., Kuipers, L. and Berkowitz, R.: 'A Trial of Social Intervention in the Families of Schizophrenic Patients', *British Journal of Psychiatry*, 141, pp. 121–34, 1982.

Berkowitz, R., Shavit, N. et al,: 'A Trial of Family Therapy Versus a Relatives Group for Schizophrenia', *British Journal of Psychiatry*, 154, pp. 58–66, 1989.

[7]Falloon, I. R. H., Boyd, J. L., McGill, C. W., Razani, J., Moss, H. B. and Gilderman, A. M.: 'Family Management in the Prevention of Exacerbation of Schizophrenia: A Controlled Study, *New England Journal of Medicine*, 306, p.1437, 1982.

Schizophrenia

Before describing the drugs used to treat serious mental illnesses, it is worth taking a closer look at the particular illness they are most used for.

Schizophrenia is a serious mental illness in which a group of experiences appear together in one person. Briefly, these symptoms or experiences are: hallucinations (sensory experiences for which no external cause exists, such as hearing voices or feeling things that are not there); delusions (irrational beliefs, such as the belief that one's thoughts are being controlled or broadcast), markedly illogical thought processes; inappropriate emotional responses; social withdrawal; blunted emotions and grossly disturbed behaviour. In the industrialized world schizophrenia is said to affect approximately one out of two hundred people. The symptoms of schizophrenia place heavy burdens on the lives of its sufferers, and the prejudices they encounter in their communities add substantially to those burdens. Nobody really knows what causes schizophrenia but research into the structure and activity of the brain, as well as into genetics, sociology and psychology, has brought promising pointers to some of its possible causes.

The experience of schizophrenia has been compared to the experience of a dream or nightmare. In a dream our minds are flooded by a jumble of thoughts and emotions which do not conform to any logical patterns; we are pitched into a world of vivid imagery in which the familiar and the strange are woven together. We may be terrified by threatening and bizarre images, sounds and feelings, or haunted by unseen menaces. We may feel ourselves to be masters of all around us, with unlimited powers to control people and events. We may hear other people's thoughts, walk on or under water, fly, or go skateboarding with the Queen Mother. We may believe ourselves to be controlled by menacing, unseen forces. Our emotions might be entirely inappropriate to the events in which we find ourselves in our dream, for example, laughing at the death of a loved one or weeping inconsolably at a moment of triumph. Dreams seldom unfold with the neat and ordered story-lines of films; in dreams the chaotic and the fantastical are as real to us as are the events around us when we are awake. Such dream states resemble the experience of schizophrenia and when experienced during a person's waking hours, they are described as 'psychotic', meaning that they come from within the person rather than being real in the world around that person. Someone who is psychotic is often described as having lost contact with reality, in contrast to someone diagnosed as neurotic, who may have irrational fears or anxieties but who remains in contact with the events and people around him or her.

Even in our waking moments we may glimpse the experience of schizophrenia. How many of us are half convinced that we can make it rain by washing the car or going out without a raincoat? This is not so far removed from a paranoid delusion.

The foundations of the modern concept of schizophrenia were laid during the latter part of the nineteenth century by one of the leading pioneers of modern psychiatry, Emil Kraepelin. He described and classified the group of symptoms as *dementia praecox*, the dementia of early life, but it was the Swiss psychiatrist Eugen Bleuler who used the term schizophrenia to denote the concept of a split mind. The work of Kraepelin and Bleuler shaped modern diagnostic conventions regarding schizophrenia.

Research into the possibility that abnormal brain chemistry is a primary cause of schizophrenia has been pursued with vigour and enthusiasm for over a century. However, much of this research has produced little more than a long litany of unfulfilled promises of imminent breakthroughs. With the use of brain scans, more recent research has identified evidence of small areas of brain atrophy in some but not all people with schizophrenia. However, although roughly a quarter of such patients have these abnormalities, similar abnormalities are seen in people who do not suffer from schizophrenia. Another approach has been to measure the responses both of people with schizophrenia and their relatives to a variety of stimuli, such as flashing lights and noises. This research indicates that sufferers from schizophrenia, along with some of their relatives, have abnormally high responses to these stimuli. These findings may be interpreted as evidence that there is a link between schizophrenia and the way in which the brain processes information, but these are speculations and there is as yet no hard evidence to confirm them.

Geneticists, on the other hand, have been searching for an abnormal or delinquent gene as a factor in causing schizophrenia, but so far researchers in this field have been less than rigorous in gathering and interpreting data. Franz Kallmann, a leading pioneer of genetic research into schizophrenia, published from the mid-thirties to the mid-fifties a series of findings from studies of twins that purported to show an overwhelming statistical link between heredity and schizophrenia. But Kallmann not only appears to have fiddled his results, but also to have kept some rather shady company in Nazi Germany, where he worked before emigrating to the USA. Kallmann's name continues to appear in learned articles and psychiatric textbooks, despite the fact that his work has been systematically rubbished and ridiculed by numerous scholarly reviewers. More recent and more rigorous studies into twins have shown that heredity may be a predisposing factor in schizophrenia. But the critics of this research argue that environmental factors, such as the twins being brought up in similar circumstances, may explain their increased susceptibility to the same mental illness.

On the socio-economic front there are some facts about the distribution of schizophrenia which seem relevant. Most of the research shows that it is much more commonly diagnosed amongst the poorer classes. Social factors have also very clearly been shown to have a major impact on the rate of relapse amongst those suffering from schizophrenia. The possibility that disturbed or confusing relationships within families may cause schizophrenia has also been suggested. Subsequent research and observation, however, has neither confirmed nor lent credibility to this theory. The concept of the 'schizogenic family' (that is, a family which causes a member to become schizophrenic) has not helped sufferers or their families. Rather it has left a legacy of guilt which may have caused some families to adopt more authoritarian attitudes than they might otherwise have had towards their mentally ill relatives. The ways in which sufferers from schizophrenia and their families interact can affect the rate at which relapses occur, and help given to those families can reduce the relapse rate. An increasing number of studies have shown not only that drugs work more effectively when given along with support to the families, but also that drugs may be given in lower doses with equal effectiveness when such support is given.

The present state of understanding is that schizophrenia is a multicausal illness, but none of the evidence is absolutely conclusive. As much as we might wish it to be otherwise, for the foreseeable future, the treatment of schizophrenia will continue to be focused around very imperfect antipsychotic drugs, if for no other reason than the fact that the pharmaceutical industry will continue to back, with its formidable financial might, that research which will protect and expand its markets. We might also wish that this bias be countered by state support for more research into the possible social and psychological causes and treatments for schizophrenia, but the treatment of mental illness has never held a high priority with any government. Like it or not, the day-to-day reality for most schizophrenia sufferers will be focused around the use or non-use of antipsychotic drugs. Consequently, the real issues that have to be addressed are how we make the best use of these drugs and the context in which they should be used. The debate over the merits of care in the community has so far been uninformed by a real understanding of the actual, rather than the assumed, effectiveness of these drugs.

Whatever its causes, mental illness occurs in a social context and has social consequences and it simply is not good enough to leave it to the doctors and the drugs they prescribe. Mental hospitals have been shown to be universities of helplessness in which psychiatrists have been the professors, but it would be naïve and misguided to close them only to set up an open university of helplessness within the community. With the honourable exception of the work of a few multidisciplinary teams, the treatment of schizophrenia in Britain is limited to the use of drugs to control its symptoms. This is the easy part of treating mental illness. The difficult part usually starts after the diagnosis and treatment, when the mentally ill person has to find or learn ways of coping with life in commuinity, which at best may be indifferent and at worst downright hostile. To get by in a community requires access to a much more complex range of skills, and many psychiatrists have struggled to create treatment services which go beyond dealing merely with symptoms. The acid test of these services is not how scientifically learned the staff are, but how acceptable the treatment would be to the man or woman in the street should they or someone they care about need them. By this test, many services fall very short of the ideal. The prospect of madness is frightening but so is the prospect of becoming a psychiatric patient. People who suffer from schizophrenia are often referred to as 'schizophrenics' as though they were members of a separate subspecies of humanity. Perhaps this is not so much a reflection of unkindness or malice as a way of distancing ourselves from those whose outward behaviour is a disturbing reminder of our own inner fears.

Six-point Guide to Getting the Most from Antipsychotic Drugs

In order to maximize the benefits and minimize the side effects of antipsychotic drugs the following points should be borne in mind:

★ Antipsychotic drugs should be used at the lowest possible dose which achieves the maximum relief of symptoms.

★ Not more than one antipsychotic drug should be used at any one time.

★ If medication to control side effects is necessary its use should be regularly reviewed and stopped as soon as possible.

★ Antipsychotic drugs should not be prescribed in combination with other psychiatric drugs unless there are compelling reasons to do so. Such combination prescribing should be subject to close and regular review and should be stopped as soon as possible.

★ Antipsychotic drugs should be used as a part of a comprehensive treatment plan which includes help to reduce stress in the daily life of the patient. For patients who live with families those families should also receive help.

★ People receiving treatment with antipsychotic drugs should be cautious in their use of alcoholic drinks.

FAST FACTS	
Purpose	The treatment of schizophrenia. Short-term control of agitation, dangerous behaviour and mania. In very low doses, the treatment of uncontrollable hiccups. In very low doses and over short periods of time, the treatment of severe anxiety.
How do I take it?	In tablet form *or* by injection *or* drunk as a syrup. People may receive antipsychotics in all these forms concurrently but this is rarely justified.

continued

When do I take it?	In tablet or syrup form, as directed by the prescribing doctor. Injections may be given in emergencies. With the long-acting or depot preparations, it may be given on a fortnightly or monthly basis.
How long does it take to work?	These drugs affect people differently and will act more rapidly for some than for others. The time a drug takes to work will vary, depending on the particular compound used, the dose and on the method of administration. When administered by injection some of the drugs' actions will occur very rapidly. When the drug is first taken it may take up to three weeks before it begins to act on symptoms.
Should I expect to experience side effects?	Yes, but some of these may be more severe when you first begin to take the drug.
What are the most common side effects?	Drowsiness; apathy; nightmares; depression; nasal congestion; trembling hands; blurred vision; sensitivity to sunlight (a risk of sunburn); impotence; reduced capacity for orgasm; changes in menstrual cycle; weight gain; reduced body temperature; reduced blood pressure; Parkinsonism. With long-term use tardive dyskinesia (see p. 160–162). NB Some of the side effects vary in severity between different compounds. For fuller details consult the individual drugs listing.
What should I do if I experience other distressing side effects?	You should always inform your doctor about side effects as it may be possible to reduce their severity by a reduction in dose or by drugs prescribed specifically to reduce these effects (see p. 165–169).

continued

How long should I continue to take it?	It may be necessry for you to continue taking this drug for years. This will depend on your condition and individual needs. You should review the dose you take and the need to continue with the drug at least every six months with the prescribing doctor.
Is it addictive?	No, but you may develop a physical dependency on the drug which may cause you to experience muscular discomfort and insomnia if you suddenly stop taking the drug. You will not develop any craving for the drug, nor will you need to increase the dose to gain its benefits.

Antipsychotic drugs are often prescribed with other medications to counter their side effects. These drugs are listed and described on pp. 165–169.

ANTIPSYCHOTIC DRUGS ARE PRESCRIBED FOR SERIOUS MENTAL ILLNESS OR DISTRESS · IT IS INADVISABLE AND POTENTIALLY HAZARDOUS TO STOP TAKING THEM AGAINST MEDICAL ADVICE AS YOU MAY EXPERIENCE A SERIOUS RECURRENCE OF THE CONDITION FOR WHICH THE DRUG WAS PRESCRIBED · IF YOU ARE WORRIED ABOUT THE EFFECTS OF THE DRUG *ALWAYS* CONSULT YOUR DOCTOR · IF YOU ARE UNABLE TO RESOLVE THE PROBLEM WITH YOUR OWN DOCTOR YOU SHOULD SEEK A SECOND MEDICAL OPINION

CHLORPROMAZINE

Trade name	Description
Largactil	10 mg, 25 mg, 50 mg and 100 mg off-white coated tablets. Clear golden-brown syrup. Orange suspension to be diluted with water. Ampoules of pale straw-coloured liquid for injection.
Chlorpromazine (generic name)	10 mg, 25 mg, 50 mg and 100 mg white coated tablets. Elixir (liquid) to be drunk as directed by doctor. Ampoules for injection. 100 mg suppositories for insertion into rectum.

General Information

Chlorpromazine was the first effective antipsychotic drug to be used in psychiatry and remains one of the most widely prescribed drugs in this group. It is the drug against which all the other antipsychotics are compared in order to measure their effectiveness and side effects. Chlorpromazine is an effective treatment for symptoms such as hallucinations, thought disorders and delusions caused by schizophrenia and other psychotic conditions. It may also be used to control violent and difficult behaviour. In common with other antipsychotic compounds it is impossible to predict the dose of Chlorpromazine an individual patient will need for the relief of symptoms. The dose level needs to be established through trial and error and by gradually increasing it until the desired effect has been achieved. It is often possible to reduce the dose once the patient's condition has been stabilized.

Chlorpromazine and its derivatives do prevent some patients from relapsing, but a significant number will relapse whilst taking them. There is also a small number of patients who will not benefit from antipsychotic drugs and some whose condition will worsen if they take them. It is not possible to predict which patients will not benefit from chlorpromazine and its derivatives; neither is it possible to predict which patients will suffer a relapse whilst taking these drugs. Evidence of a

Dosage Information

Adult (16 and over): For the control of schizophrenia and other psychoses, serious agitation, over-excitement or violent and dangerous behaviour. *By mouth*: treatment begins with 25 mg three times per day or a single dose of 75 mg at night. This dose may be increased according to the response of the patient to a normal maintenance dose of between 75 mg and 300 mg per day. Occasionally, in the case of severe symptoms, the daily dose may be increased to 1000 mg per day. Doses which exceed this are controversial.

Dose by deep intramuscular injection: For the relief of very severe symptoms. 25–50 mg every six to eight hours.

Dose by rectum: 100 mg suppositories every six to eight hours.

Elderly and physically frail: One-third to a half of the normal adult dose. Elderly people are more prone to side effects and to suffering from tardive dyskinesia (see p. 160-2).

Children: Between the ages of one to five, 500 micrograms per kilo of the child's body weight. Between the ages of six and twelve, one-third to half the adult dose. The use of antipsychotic drugs for children is controversial.

Side Effects and Further Information

Chlorpromazine causes more sedation and drowsiness than other antipsychotic compounds (see pp. 157–162 for a full description of side effects).

Prolonged use may cause tardive dyskinesia, a condition which causes people to develop facial tics and other involuntary movements (for a fuller description of tardive dyskinesia and its side effects, see pp. 160–2).

Caution is advised in handling liquid forms of chlorpromazine as it can cause unpleasant skin reactions.

BENPERIDOL

Trade name	Description
Anquil	250 microgram white tablets marked JANSEN on one side and 0.25 on the other.

General Information

An antipsychotic drug whose manufacturers claim is useful in the control of deviant and antisocial sexual behaviour. It has been advertised for its ability to suppress masturbation in people with learning difficulties. A very controversial drug whose value according to the British National Formulary 'is not established.'

Dosage Information

Adult (16 and over): Between 0.25–1.5 mg daily in divided doses.

Elderly and physically frail: Treatment begins with half the adult dose.

Children: Benperidol should not be used to treat children.

Side Effects and Further Information

If benperidol has any place in the treatment of mental illness it is a very limited one. It is not as sedating as chlorpromazine and more often causes inner agitation, physical restlessness, a mask-like facial appearance, tremors, and muscular rigidity.

CLOZAPINE	
Trade name	*Description*
Clozaril	25 mg yellow scored tablets. 100 mg yellow scored tablets (for use in hospitals only).

General Information

Clozapine is only prescribed when a patient cannot tolerate, or his or her symptoms are not relieved by, another antipsychotic drug. It can cause agranulocytosis, a serious and potentially fatal blood disorder which causes damage to the bone marrow. For this reason its use is restricted to prescribers, pharmacists and patients registered with the Clozaril Patient Monitoring Group. Before Clozapine is used the patient's blood must be tested for any existing disorder. During the first 18 weeks of treatment the patient's blood should be tested every week to monitor any changes caused by the drug. Thereafter a blood test is necessary every two weeks. If any signs of blood disorder occur the drug should be withdrawn.

Clozapine should be used with extreme caution in patients with infections, liver or kidney disorders, epilepsy, heart disease, enlarged prostate gland, glaucoma (a condition in which there is abnormal pressure in the eye) and paralytic ileus (an obstruction in the intestines).

Dosage Information

Adult (16 and over): Treatment begins with 25–50 mg per day which may be increased or decreased according to the response of the patient. If a larger dose is necessary this should be done by increasing the dose by 125–50 mg per day (for elderly people, by 25 mg) over a period of seven to fourteen days, to reach 300 mg per day) the drug may be taken as a single dose at bedtime. The usual dose for psychotic symptoms is between 200–450 mg per day (**a maximum dose of 900 mg per day**), which should be reduced to a usual maintenance dose of between 150–300 mg per day.

Children: Clozapine should not be used to treat children.

Side Effects and Further Information

Clozapine may cause potentially fatal blood disorders, the symptoms of which are fever and ulcerations of the mouth and throat which may rapidly lead to collapse and death. Clozapine should be avoided by people with a history of drug-caused blood disorders, bone marrow disorders and epilepsy. It should be avoided in people who have become psychotic as a result of drug or alcohol abuse, coma and depression.

Clozapine should not be taken during pregnancy or whilst breast-feeding.

The side effects of clozapine include: Excessive salivation. Periods when the mouth is very dry. Reduced blood pressure which may cause patients to feel faint when they stand. Physical and psychological restlessness. Increased body temperature. Tremors. Inner feelings of agitation. Drowsiness. Blurred vision. Muscular rigidity and a mask-like facial appearance. An increase in the risk of suffering epileptic fits.

Rare side effects include: Arrhythmia (changes in the heart rate, palpitations, breathlessness and chest pains). Delirium. Liver disease. Neuroleptic malignant syndrome (a rare and potentially fatal condition caused by antipsychotic drugs, the symptoms of which are an increase in body temperature, sweating, jerky involuntary movements of the limbs, drowsiness, rapid breathing, stupor, and coma).

DROPERIDOL	
Trade name	Description
Droleptan	10 mg yellow tablets marked JANSSEN on one side and D over 10 on the other. Clear liquid to be taken orally. Ampoules for injection.

General Information

Droperidol is used to boost the effects of pain-relieving drugs in surgery as a premedication and as a treatment for post-operative nausea. It is also used to treat the side effects of nausea and vomiting caused by drugs used in the treatment of cancer. In psychiatry it is used to calm agitated, manic and psychotic patients. Its effects are identical to those of haloperidol. In this guide only information about droperidol's use in psychiatry is given.

Dosage Information

Adult (16 and over): For sedation and emergency control of mania. *By mouth*: 5–10 mg repeated every four to six hours as necessary.

By injection: Up to 10 mg repeated every four to six hours as necessary.

Elderly and physically frail: Treatment begins with half the adult dose.

Children: 0.5–1 mg per day, which if necessary should be increased with care. The use of anitpsychotic drugs in children is controversial and should be avoided if possible.

Side Effects and Further Information

Droperidol is less sedating than chlorpromazine but more often causes inner agitation, physical restlessness, a mask-like facial appearance, tremors and muscular rigidity. Prolonged use may cause tardive dyskinesia, a condition which causes facial tics and other involuntary movements (for a fuller description of tardive dyskinesia and its side effects, see pp. 160–2).

FLUPENTHIXOL	
Trade name	*Description*
Depixol	3 mg yellow tablets printed with Lundbeck on one side. Straw-coloured liquid in ampoule, vial or syringe, to be injected.

General Information

Flupenthixol is a potent and rapidly acting antipsychotic which may be administered by daily doses or given as an injection which will last for between two and four weeks (see flupenthixol decanoate, p. 149). When given as a daily treatment it is relatively short-acting. It is said to have an alerting effect on withdrawn patients, which may be related to the feelings of restlessness which is a common side effect of this particular group of antipsychotic drugs.

Dosage Information

Adult (16 and over): Treatment begins with 3–9 mg twice daily, increased or decreased according to the response of the patient. **The maximum dose is 18 mg (six 3 mg tablets) per day.**

Elderly and phsycially frail: Should be avoided for the treatment of elderly, confused or senile people.

Children: The manufacturers recommend that flupenthixol should not be used to treat children.

Side Effects and Further Information

In approximately 25 per cent of patients flupenthixol causes extrapyramidal side effects: inner agitation, physical restlessness, a mask-like facial appearance, tremors and muscular rigidity. Prolonged use may cause tardive dyskinesia, a condition which causes facial tics and other involuntary movements (for a fuller description of tardive dyskinesia and its side effects, see pp. 160–2).

FLUPHENAZINE HYDROCHLORIDE	
Trade name	*Description*
Moditen	1 mg pink tablets. 2.5 mg yellow tablets. 5 mg white tablets.

General Information

Fluphenazine is a potent antipsychotic drug used to control the symptoms of schizophrenia, extreme agitation, withdrawal, dangerous behaviour and mania. It is said to be particularly useful in treating paranoid psychosis. It may be given as a daily dose or as a depot injection lasting from ten days to three weeks (see fluphenazine enanthate, p. 152). It is more likely to cause extrapyramidal side effects (see below) than some other antipsychotic compounds.

Dosage Information

Adult (16 and over): For anxiety and non-psychotic behaviour disturbances. 1 mg twice daily, increased if necessary to 2 mg twice daily.

For schizophrenia psychotic withdrawal, mania and paranoid psychosis. Treatment begins with between 2.5–10 mg per day in two or three doses, depending on the severity of the symptoms. The dose may be increased or decreased according to the response of the patient. **The maximum dose is 20 mg per day**. Higher doses should only be given with great caution.

Elderly and physically frail: As elderly people are more likely to suffer from side effects they should be treated with lower doses. Doses above 10 mg per day should only be used with great caution in elderly people.

Children: The manufacturers recommend that fluphenazine should not be used to treat children.

Side Effects and Further Information

Fluphenazine should be avoided in comatose patients and patients who suffer from diseased blood vessels in the brain; phaeochromocytoma (a tumour in the adrenal gland which causes increased blood pressure and heart rate, palpitations and headaches); liver disease; kidney disease; heart disease; or severe depression.

Fluphenazine is less sedating than chlorpromazine but it is more likely to cause extrapyramidal side effects (inner agitation, physical restlessness, a mask-like facial appearance, tremors and muscular rigidity). Prolonged use may cause tardive dyskinesia, a condition which causes facial tics and other involuntary movements (for a fuller description of tardive dyskinesia see pp. 160–2).

HALOPERIDOL

Trade name	Description
Dozic	Liquid to be taken orally.
Fortunan	0.5 mg white tablets. 1.5 mg white tablets. 5 mg green tablets. 10 mg pink tablets. 20 mg white tablets.
Haldol	5 mg blue tablets. 10 mg yellow tablets. Liquid to be taken orally.
Haloperidol (generic name)	1.5 mg, 5 mg, 10 mg and 20 mg white tablets.
Serenace	0.5 mg green capsules. 1.5 mg pink tablets. 10 mg pale pink tablets. 20 mg dark pink tablets. Liquid to be taken orally. Ampoules for injection.

General Information

Haloperidol is a highly potent antipsychotic which can act rapidly to control the symptoms of schizophrenia, mania and dangerous behaviour. It is less sedating than chlorpromazine but its other side effects may be more severe and more frequent. In particular the side effects which give the patient a zombie-like appearance and cause physical and psychological restlessness and depression are more common.

Dosage Information

Adult (16 and over): For the control of the symptoms of schizophrenia, mania, extreme agitation and dangerous behaviour. *By mouth*: Treatment begins with between 1.5–20 mg per day in divided doses, gradually increased or decreased according to the response of the patient. **The maximum dose is 100 mg, occasionally 200 mg per day** in very disturbed patients.

By injection: 2–10 mg, increasing to 30 mg for emergency control, then repeated injections of 5 mg every four to eight hours. In extreme circumstances the injections may be given hourly until control of the symptoms has been achieved.

Elderly and physically frail: Half the adult starting dose, to **a maximum dose of 4 mg per day**.

Children: *By mouth*: 0.025–0.05 mg per kilogram of body weight daily, to **a maximum dose of 10 mg daily**; or for adolescents (13–16) up to **a maximum dose of 30 mg**. In *exceptional* circumstances up to 60 mg per day may be given. The administration of haloperidol by injection to children is *not* recommended. The use of antipsychotic drugs to treat children is controversial.

Side Effects and Further Information

Haloperidol is less sedating than chlorpromazine but is more likely to cause extrapyramidal side effects (inner agitation, physical restlessness, a mask-like facial appearance, tremors and muscular rigidity). Prolonged use may cause tardive dyskinesia, a condition which causes facial tics and other involuntary movements (for a fuller description of tardive dyskinesia see pp. 160–2).

LOXAPINE	
Trade name	*Description*
Loxapac	10 mg yellow and green capsules. 25 mg light green and dark green capsules. 50 mg blue and dark green capsules.

Dosage Information

Loxapine is used for the treatment of schizophrenia, mania and other psychotic states. It must be used (if at all) with great caution in patients with heart disease as most patients who take this drug will experience an increased pulse rate. Loxapine must also be used with great caution – if at all – in patients prone to suffering epileptic fits as it can cause fits, even if anticonvulsant drugs are being taken. Loxapine is more dangerous in overdose than other antipsychotic drugs and is described in the British National Formulary as having 'a high potential for serious neurological and cardiac toxicity'. It is said to cause less drowsiness than other antipsychotics.

Dosage Information

Adult (16 and over): Treatment begins with 20–50 mg per day taken in two divided doses, which may be increased if necessary over a period of seven to ten days to 60–100 mg daily. In the higher dose range the drug may be taken in three or four divided doses per day. **The maximum dose is 250 mg per day**, which should be reduced to a more normal maintenance dose range of 20–100 mg per day.

Children: Loxapine is not recommended for the treatment of children.

Side Effects and Further Information

Loxapine is similar in its effects to other antipsychotics and may cause weight gain or weight loss, nausea and vomiting, laboured or difficult breathing, blurred vision, trembling limbs, inner restlessness, flushing and headaches. Prolonged use may cause tardive dyskinesia, a condition which causes facial tics and other involuntary movements (for a fuller description of tardive dyskinesia and its side effects, see pp. 160–2).

METHOTRIMEPRAZINE	
Trade name	*Description*
Nozanan	25 mg white tablets. Ampoules for injection.

General Information

Used in the treatment of schizophrenia, mania and other psychotic states, the main differences between methotrimeprazine and chlorpromazine are its price and its sedating effects. It costs three times as much as chlorpromazine and it is more likely to cause drowsiness, weakness and apathy.

Dosage Information

Adult (16 and over): For schizophrenia and psychotic conditions. *By mouth*: Treatment begins with 25–50 mg per day which may be increased or decreased according to the response of the patient. Hospital in-patients may start treatment at between 100–200 mg per day in three divided doses, to be increased or decreased according to the response of the patient. **The maximum dose is 1000 mg per day**. Patients receiving high doses should be kept in bed. When symptoms have been stabilized the dose should be adjusted downward to the minimum dose which controls the symptoms.

Elderly and physically frail: Methotrimeprazine should not be given to people over the age of 50 unless the risk to the patient of a serious reduction in blood pressure has been assessed. Patients with heart problems may be at risk of potentially dangerous effects.

Children: Children are more likely than adults to suffer from the powerful sedating effects of methotrimeprazine. The use of doses by mouth exceeding 40 mg per day is not recommended by the manufacturers. The usual maintenance dose for a ten-year-old child is said to be between 15 and 20 mg. The use of antipsychotic drugs to treat children is controversial.

Side Effects and Further Information

Methotrimeprazine is also used in the care of terminally ill patients to reduce restlessness and agitation, to increase the effectiveness of pain-relieving drugs and to reduce vomiting. It may cause weight gain or weight loss, nausea and vomiting, laboured or difficult breathing, blurred vision, trembling limbs, inner restlessness, flushing and headaches. Prolonged use may cause tardive dyskinesia, a condition which causes facial tics and other involuntary movements (for a fuller description of tardive dyskinesia and its side effects, see pp. 160–2).

OXYPERTINE	
Trade name	*Description*
Integrin	10 mg white capsules. 40 mg speckled white tablets.

General Information

In low doses oxypertine is promoted for the short-term treatment of anxiety and depression. In higher doses it is promoted as a treatment for the symptoms of schizophrenia, mania, other psychotic states and the short-term control of behavioural disturbances. It is claimed to be particularly relevant to the needs of withdrawn schizophrenic patients. In low doses oxypertine is said to cause agitation and hyperactivity and in high doses sedation. In general its effects are broadly similar to chlorpromazine.

Dosage Information

Adult (16 and over): *For the short-term treatment of severe anxiety and depression.* Treatment begins with 10 mg three to four times per day after meals, which may be increased or decreased according to the response of the patient. **The maximum dose is 60 mg (six tablets) per day.**

For the treatment of schizophrenia, the short-term management of problem behaviour arising from mental illness and other psychotic states. Treatment begins with 80–120 mg (two or three tablets) per day, which may be increased or decreased according to the response of the patient. **The maximum dose is 300 mg per day.** When control of the symptoms has been achieved the dose should be reduced to the minimum necessary to control the symptoms.

Elderly and physically frail: Doses lower than the normal range of adult doses are recommended.

Children: There are no dose recommendations for children. The use of antipsychotic drugs to treat children is controversial.

Side Effects and Further Information

Oxypertine is broadly similar to chlorpromazine in its actions but is said to cause extrapyramidal side effects less frequently. Prolonged use may cause tardive dyskinesia, a condition which causes facial tics and other involuntary movements (for a fuller description of tardive dyskinesia and its side effects, see pp. 160–2).

PERICYAZINE	
Trade name	*Description*
Neulactil	2.5 mg yellow tablets marked Neulactil 2.5. 10 mg yellow tablets marked Neulactil 10. 25 mg yellow tablets marked Neulactil 25. Brown syrup to be taken orally.

General Information

Pericyazine is promoted for the treatment of schizophrenia, mania, other psychotic conditions and for the control of problem behaviour in adults and children. Its effects are broadly similar to those of chlorpromazine but it is more likely to cause drowsiness and apathy. At the beginning of treatment reduced blood pressure is common and this may cause patients to feel faint.

Dosage Information

Adult: *For the short-term treatment of anxiety, agitation and problem behaviour.* Treatment begins with 15–30 mg per day in two divided doses, the higher dose taken at bedtime, to be increased or decreased according to the patient's response.

For the treatment of schizophrenia, mania and other psychotic states. Treatment begins with 75 mg in divided doses which may be increased if necessary by adding 25 mg to the daily dose at weekly intervals. **The usual maximum dose is 300 mg per day**.

Elderly and physically frail: *For the short-term treatment of severe anxiety.* Treatment begins with 5–10 mg per day divided into two doses the larger dose taken at bedtime.

For the treatment of schizophrenia, mania and other psychotic states. Treatment begins with 15–30 mg per day which may be increased or decreased according to the response of the patient. Half or quarter the normal adult maintenance dose may be adequate.

Children: *For the control of serious behavioural problems arising from mental illness only.* Treatment begins with 0.5 mg per day for a child with a body weight of 10 kilograms, increased by 1 mg for each additional 5 kilograms of body weight. The dose may be increased or decreased according to the response of the child. The maximum daily dose of 10 mg may be gradually increased but should not exceed twice the starting dose. The use of antipsychotic drugs to treat children is controversial.

Side Effects and Further Information

Pericyazine is more sedating than chlorpromazine and frequently causes a reduction in blood pressure which may cause the patient to feel faint when standing, particularly at the beginning of treatment. Prolonged use may cause tardive dyskinesia, a condition which causes facial tics and other involuntary movements (for a fuller description of tardive dyskinesia and its side effects, see pp. 160–2).

PERPHENAZINE

Trade name	Description
Fentazin	2 mg white tablets marked AH/1C. 4 mg white tablets marked AH/2C.

General Information

Perphenazine is used to treat the symptoms of serious mental illnesses such as schizophrenia, mania and other psychotic states of mind. In comparison with chlorpromazine it is said to cause less sedation but much more severe extrapyramidal effects such as muscle spasms in the neck, shoulders and trunk, blurred vision, dry mouth, stomach upsets and restlessness. Because of the severity of these side effects the drug's manufacturers tell doctors that it should not be used to treat children below the age of 14 or agitated and restless elderly people.

Dosage Information

Adult (16 and over): For the treatment of schizophrenia, mania, psychotic states and the control of problem behaviour. Treatment begins with 4 mg three times per day which may be increased or decreased depending on the response of the patient. If necessary the dose can be increased under close supervision to **a maximum dose of 24 mg per day**.

Elderly and physically frail: A quarter to half the normal adult starting dose is suggested by the manufacturers.

Children: Perphenazine should not be given to children below the age of 14. The use of antipsychotic drugs to treat children is controversial.

Side Effects and Further Information

Perphenazine is in the same group of antipsychotic drugs as haloperidol, which is more often prescribed. In very low doses it may be used for the treatment of vomiting and nausea. Prolonged use may cause tardive dyskinesia, a condition which causes facial tics and other involuntary movements (for a fuller description of tardive dyskinesia and its side effects, see pp. 160–2).

PIMOZIDE	
Trade name	*Description*
Orap	2 mg white tablets marked JANSSEN. 4 mg pale green tablets marked JANSSEN. 10 mg white tablets marked JANSSEN.

General Information

Pimozide is one of the newer antipsychotic drugs, having been introduced in Britain in 1971. It is used to treat the same range of symptoms as the other drugs in this class and is suggested to be useful in the treatment of 'monosymptomatic hypochondriacal psychosis'. In other words, for people who believe that they are ill although doctors are unable to find anything wrong with them.

In August the Government drug watchdog organization, the Committee on Safety of Medicines (CSM), issued a report to doctors drawing their attention to the possible risk of patients taking pimozide being exposed to heart damage. Thirteen sudden and unexpected deaths of patients taking the drug have been reported. Seven of these patients were between the ages of 13 and 17. Five of the 13 patients were also taking other antipsychotic drugs (polypharmacy) and ten were receiving more than the normal recommended maintenance dose. In their report the Committee suggests that prior to the drug being taken, patients should be given electrocardiographical (ECG) tests to ensure that their hearts are sufficiently robust to receive the drug. Patients receiving in excess of 16 mg per day should regularly have ECG heart checks. The report also warns doctors that the risk of heart damage may be greater if pimozide is used with other antipsychotic drugs. It recommends that substantially lower doses of pimozide should be used than those recommended in the prescribers' handbooks. The doses given below are those recommended in the CSM report.

Dosage Information

Adult (16 and over): Treatment with pimozide begins with a dose of between 2–4 mg per day, except in the short-term management of very serious symptoms when the starting dose may be increased to as much as 10 mg per day. If necessary the dose can be raised in steps of 2–4 mg daily to **the maximum daily dose of 20 mg**.

Elderly and physically frail: Pimozide has a long half-life (see below) and elderly people who regularly take it may be prone to levels of the drug building up in their bodies and reaching unintentionally high doses. This exposes elderly people to increased risks of distressing and potentially dangerous side effects, and increases their exposure to the long-term hazards of antipsychotic drugs. The manufacturers recommend that elderly patients should be treated with half the normal starting dose for adults.

Children: Not recommended for the treatment of children.

Side Effects and Further Information

Pimozide has a long 'half-life', which means that it remains in the body of the patient for a longer time than other similar drugs. This long 'half-life' is not predictable from patient to patient. In some patients the half-life of pimozide is 55 hours whilst for others it is more than 150 hours. When the drug stays in the system for a long period, the patient will begin to accumulate quantities of the drug in the body, which in some patients can lead to overdoses being gradually built up.

Prolonged use may cause tardive dyskinesia, a condition which causes involuntary movements of the mouth, face, shoulders, trunk and limbs (for a fuller description of tardive dyskinesia see pp. 160–2).

PROCHLORPERAZINE

Trade name	Description
Buccastem (low-dose preparation for treating vertigo, nausea and vomiting)	3 mg pale yellow tablets.
Prochlorperazine (generic name)	5 mg white tablets.
Stemetil	5 mg off-white tablets marked Stemetil 5. 25 mg off-white tablets marked Stemetil 25. Injection. 5 mg and 25 mg suppositories. Syrup.
Vertigon (low-dose preparation for treating vertigo, nausea and vomiting)	10 mg clear capsules with purple top marked No 4. 15 mg clear capsules with yellow top marked No 5.

General Information

Prochlorperazine in low-dose preparations is recommended for the treatment of 'labrinthitis, and for nausea and vomiting from whatever cause including that associated with migraine, *schizophrenia (particularly in the chronic stage), acute mania and as an adjunct to the short-term management of anxiety'* (author's italics). In high-dose preparations it is recommended for the treatment of *'schizophrenia and other psychotic disorders'* (author's italics). This is confusing, as it appears to suggest to prescribers that they give high doses of the drug to treat patients suffering with schizophrenia and other psychotic conditions, and low doses of the same drug to treat those same patients for the nausea and vomiting that are 'associated' with them.

As an antipsychotic drug, prochlorperazine is said to be less sedating than chlorpromazine but to have more serious dystonic effects such as muscular spasms in the neck, shoulders and trunk, rigidity and tremors.

Dosage Information

Adult (16 and over): *For the treatment of labrinthitis, vertigo, nausea and vomiting. By mouth:* 5 mg three times per day which may be increased if necessary to **a maximum dose of 30 mg per day**, which may then be gradually reduced to between 5–10 mg per day.

By injection: 12.5 mg injection followed by tablets or syrup after six hours if necessary.

By rectum: 25 mg suppository followed after six hours by tablets or syrup.

For the treatment of the symptoms of schizophrenia, mania and other psychotic conditions. By mouth: Treatment begins with 12.5 mg twice daily, increased if necessary in steps of 12.5 mg daily and in intervals of between four and twelve days to **the maximum daily dose per day of 75–100 mg**. The dose given may be higher than the maximum in a minority of patients but once the maximum control of symptoms has been achieved the dose should be reduced to the minimum possible to control symptoms.

By injection: Between 12.5 mg and 25 mg twice or three times per day.

By rectum: Suppositories of between 12.5 mg and 25 mg per day, to be changed to tablets or syrup as soon as possible.

Elderly and physically frail: Elderly patients should be started at a lower than normal adult dose. Caution is advised in treating the elderly with this drug as they are more prone to suffer distressing side effects and are more vulnerable to the long-term hazards of antipsychotic drugs.

Children: Prochlorperazine should not be used to treat mental illness in children but in very low doses given in tablet or syrup form it may be used with caution for children with a body weight greater than 10 kilograms, to prevent nausea and vomiting. The manufacturers recommend a dose rate of 0.025 mg per kilogram of body weight per day. With doses of 0.5 mg per kilogram of the child's body weight great caution is recommended because of serious dystonic side effects (see above under General Information). Prochlorperazine should not be given to children under 10 kilograms body weight and should not be administered to any child by injection.

Side Effects and Further Information

Prochlorperazine has been used as an anti-emetic and antipsychotic drug for many years. It has no obvious advantages over the many similar drugs in this group. In the decision of which of the antipsychotics to use, the side effects are usually the deciding factor. Prolonged use may cause tardive dyskinesia, a condition which causes involuntary movements of the mouth, face, shoulders, trunk and limbs (for a fuller description of tardive dyskinesia see pp. 160–2).

SULPIRIDE

Trade name	Description
Dolmatil	200 mg white tablets marked D200.
Sulpitil	200 mg white tablets marked L113.

General Information

Sulpiride is chemically different from the other antipsychotic drugs used to treat schizophrenia and other disturbed states of mind and has a number of important differences in its range of effects and side effects. Sulpiride is said by its manufacturers to have antidepressant as well as antipsychotic effects. Where other antipsychotics often make withdrawn patients suffering from schizophrenia even more withdrawn, sulpiride can have the opposite effect of making them more alert. The condition of some seriously agitated 'hypomanic' patients may be aggravated by sulpiride and caution is recommended by the manufacturers with such patients. The risk may be greater if the patient is also taking other medications specifically for the side effects of antipsychotic drugs (for a description of drugs used to treat side effects, see pp. 165-9). Animal research has indicated that the long-term use of sulpiride may be linked to an increased incidence of benign and malignant tumours in the endocrine system. But there is no evidence as yet that such tumours are caused in man.

Dosage Information

Adult (16 and over): For patients who are floridly psychotic with hallucinations, thought disorders, delusions, inappropriate emotions and strange fixed ideas. Treatment begins with 400–800 mg per day taken in two divided doses in the morning and early evening (two or four tablets per day). This may be increased to **the maximum dose of 1200 mg twice daily**. Doses higher than this have not been shown to have any advantages for patients.

For patients who are withdrawn, apathetic, emotionally flat and depressed. Treatment begins with 400 mg twice daily (two tablets in the morning and two in the early evening). If this dose is reduced to 200 mg, the 'alerting' effect is said to be increased.

For patients with a mixture of both sets of symptoms listed above the manufacturers recommend a normal dose range of 400–600 mg per day.

Elderly and physically frail: Similar doses to the normal adult doses are recommended but caution is advised in patients with liver disorders.

Children: No dosage recommendations are made for children as there is not enough clinical evidence available upon which to base any such recommendations. The use of antipsychotic drugs to treat children is controversial.

Side Effects and Further Information

Sulpiride is one of the most recently introduced antipsychotic drugs, is less sedating than chlorpromazine, and, it is claimed, has fewer and less severe side effects. Sulpiride is less likely to affect the heart than other drugs and does not increase the risk of epileptic fits in people prone to suffering them. Prolonged use may cause tardive dyskinesia, a condition which causes involuntary movements of the mouth, face, shoulders, trunk and limbs (for a fuller description of tardive dyskinesia see pp. 160–2).

THIORIDAZINE

Trade name	Description
Melleril	10 mg white tablets marked 10. 25 mg white tablets marked 25. 50 mg white tablets marked 50. 100 mg white tablets marked 100. 25 mg per 5 ml spoon creamy-white liquid 100 mg per 5 ml spoon creamy-white liquid 25 mg per 5 ml spoon orange syrup.
Thioridazine (generic name)	10 mg white tablets. 25 mg white tablets. 50 mg white tablets. 100 mg white tablets.

General Information

Thioridazine is used to control the symptoms of schizophrenia, mania, extreme agitation and problem behaviour. It is similar in its effects to chlorpromazine but is less sedating. It should be used with caution in depressed patients as it can aggravate depression. Thioridazine should be avoided in patients who suffer from porphyria, a rare inherited disorder which affects the blood and causes a range of symptoms, such as sensitivity to sunlight, inflammation of the nerves, stomach pain and mental disturbances.

Dosage Information

Adult (16 and over): For schizophrenia, mania and psychotic states. Treatment begins with 200 mg and may be increased to **the maximum dose of 800 mg per day for hospital in-patients under close specialist supervision**. This high dose should not be given for periods longer than four weeks.

For the control of extreme agitation and dangerous behaviour. Doses between 75–200 mg may be given.

Elderly and physically frail: For the control of agitated restlessness. Between 30–100 mg per day. Caution is necessary in treating elderly people with antipsychotics, particularly patients who suffer from kidney or liver disease.

Children: Under the age of five, 1 mg per kilogram of body weight daily. Children over the age of five, between 75–300 mg per day to **a maximum dose of 300 mg per day**. The use of antipsychotic drugs to treat children is controversial.

Side Effects and Further Information

Thioridazine is a phenothiazine antipsychotic which quite commonly causes reduced blood pressure, making people feel faint. Unlike chlorpromazine, the first drug in this group, thioridazine does not carry a risk of causing jaundice. Prolonged use may cause tardive dyskinesia, a condition which causes involuntary movements of the mouth, face, shoulders, trunk and limbs (for a fuller description of tardive dyskinesia see pp. 160–2).

TRIFLUOPERAZINE

Trade name	Description
Stelazine	1 mg blue tablets marked SKF. 2 mg clear capsules with yellow caps marked 2. 5 mg blue tablets marked SKF. 10 mg clear capsules with yellow caps marked 10. 15 mg clear capsules with yellow caps marked 15. 1 mg per 5 ml spoon pale yellow peach-flavoured syrup. Pale yellow peach-flavoured concentrate containing 10 mg per 1 ml of concentrate. Ampoules for injection.
Trifluoperazine (generic name)	1 mg white tablets. 5 mg white tablets.

General Information

Trifluoperazine is a potent antipsychotic used to control the symptoms of schizophrenia, mania and other psychotic conditions. Its manufacturers claim that it is particularly useful in controlling symptoms described as 'manic' (extreme excitement and agitation). The manufacturers recommend low doses of trifluoperazine for the treatment of depression and anxiety states as it may increase depression rather than relieve it. In common with the other antipsychotics of its type, haloperidol and fluphenazine, trifluoperazine may cause more frequent and more serious extrapyramidal effects: mask-like facial expression, stiffening and trembling of the limbs, pill-rolling movements of the fingers, physical and psychological restlessness, and, occasionally, facial grimaces, an involuntary twisting motion of the neck, and rolling of the eyes. These effects may be treated with other drugs (see p. 165–9).

Dosage Information

Adult (16 and over): *Low dose.* For the short-term treatment of 'anxiety states, depressive symptoms secondary to anxiety, and agitation.' Whatever this says, trifluoperazine may cause these very symptoms. Low-dose treatment begins with 2–4 mg per day given in two doses, morning and early evening. The dose may be increased if necessary to **a maximum dose of 6 mg per day**. At doses higher than this the side effects are likely to be a bigger problem than the one for which the drug was prescribed in the first place.

High dose. For the control of the symptoms of schizophrenia, mania, other psychotic states, the control of severe agitation and problem behaviour. *By mouth*: For physically fit adults treatment begins with 10 mg per day, which can be increased if necessary after one week to 15 mg per day and may be further increased in 5 mg steps at three-day intervals until the symptoms are controlled. When the desired results have been achieved the dose should be gradually reduced to the minimum which provides relief for the patient. **There is no maximum daily dose recommended** by the manufacturers or the publishers of the British National Formulary.

By injection: Treatment begins with 1–3 mg per day given in two doses. If necessary, the dose may be increased to **a maximum dose of 6 mg per day**. When given by injection the effects and side effects of trifluoperazine are much more rapid and intense. The treatment should be changed from injection to tablets or syrup as soon as possible.

Elderly and physically frail: Treatment should begin with less than half the normal starting dose for fit adults.

Children: *Low dose*. Children aged between three and five, up to 1 mg per day. Children aged between six and twelve, up to **a maximum dose of 4 mg per day**.

High dose. By mouth: Children under 12 should not receive more than **the maximum dose of 5 mg per day in divided doses**. Should higher dose be considered necessary any increase should be based on an evaluation of the severity of the symptoms being treated and the state of health and body weight of the child. The increase should be done in steps of three-day intervals.

By injection: The administration of this drug by injection to children is not common. The manufacturers suggest that doses should be determined on the basis of 1 mg per day per 20 kilograms of the child's body weight. The use of antipsychotic drugs to treat children is controversial.

Side Effects and Further Information

Trifluoperazine is often prescribed in low doses for the treatment of confusion and agitation in the elderly. Even in very low doses some patients experience Parkinsonism, trembling hands, a shuffling walk, an expressionless face and difficulty in movement. Prolonged use may cause tardive dyskinesia, a condition which causes involuntary movements of the mouth, face, shoulders, trunk and limbs (for a fuller description of tardive dyskinesia see pp. 160–2).

TRIFLUPERIDOL	
Trade name	*Description*
Triperidol	0.5 mg white tablets marked 0.5. 1 mg white tablets marked т over 1.

General Information

Trifluperidol is one of the most powerful antipsychotic drugs used to control the symptoms of schizophrenia, mania, other psychotic states and for the control of problem behaviour. It is chemically related to haloperidol, trifluoperazine and fluphenazine. The effects and side effects of trifluperidol are similar to those of its chemical cousins but may be more severe. Occasionally patients receiving the drug will experience painful muscle spasms which the manufacturers recommend may be treated with chlorpromazine. The side effects of trifluoperidol may last for up to thee months after the drug has been withdrawn. In view of its potency and the severity of its side effects this drug should be used with great caution and sensitivity to the subjective effects of the drug on the patient.

Dosage Information

Adult (16 and over): Treatment begins with 0.5 mg daily, increased every three or four days to **the maximum daily dose of 6–8 mg per day**. In emergencies a high dose of 3 mg may be given at the start of the treatment. It is recommended that medication for the control of side effects be given concurrently with trifluperidol as severe side effects are likely to occur (for details, see pp. 165–9).

Elderly and physically frail: No dose recommendations are given but in view of the severity and frequency of side effects great caution is obviously called for in considering whether this drug is advisable.

Children: For children between the ages of five and twelve, 0.25 mg per day, increased if necessary to **a maximum dose of 2 mg per day**. The use of antipsychotic drugs to treat children is controversial.

Side Effects and Further Information

If trifluperidol is used to treat patients over long periods of time it is recommended that regular blood and liver tests are carried out. This drug should not be used in pregnancy or to treat patients prone to suffering from epileptic fits. Prolonged use may cause tardive dyskinesia, a condition which causes involuntary movements of the mouth, face, shoulders, trunk and limbs (for a fuller description of tardive dyskinesia see pp. 160–2).

ZUCLOPENTHIXOL DIHYDROCHLORIDE

Trade name	Description
Clopixol	2 mg pink tablets. 10 mg light brown tablets. 25 mg brown tablets.

General Information

Zuclopenthixol is a potent, rapidly acting antipsychotic drug used for to control the symptoms of schizophrenia, mania and other psychotic states and for the emergency control of dangerous behaviour. Particularly in the early stages of treatment the side effects may be severe. The side effects include lethargy, depression, loss of motivation, musclar rigidity and tremors. Where necessary these side effects may be reduced by other medications (for details of medication for side effects, see pp. 165–9). Zuclopenthixol may be given as a depot injection (see zuclopenthixol decanoate, p. 156).

Dosage Information

Adult: Treatment begins with 20–30 mg per day which may be increased to a maximum dose of 150 mg per day in divided doses. The usual maintenance dose is between 20–50 mg per day which should be reduced if possible.

Elderly: Lower doses should be considered in elderly or frail people.

Children: Not recommended for the treatment of children.

Side Effects and Further Information

Zuclopenthixol should not be used in the treatment of withdrawn or apathetic patients. Prolonged use may cause tardive dyskinesia, a condition which causes involuntary movements of the mouth, face, shoulders, trunk and limbs (for a fuller description of tardive dyskinesia see pp. 160–2).

Antipsychotic Depot Injections

The compounds described in this section are used to treat patients who may be reluctant or who forget to take their antipsychotic drugs. The drugs may be injected on a weekly, fortnightly, three-weekly or monthly basis. As it is often difficult to establish the dose which gives the individual the maximum relief of symptoms with the minimum of side effects, great care and sensitivity should be exercised in the use of these preparations. Sadly, there is evidence that such care is not always taken. Some depot injection clinics are merely production lines requiring the minimum effort for the nurses and psychiatrists who work in them. This is community care out of a syringe and has more in common with battery farming than with services designed to respond to the complex and changing needs of vulnerable human beings.

Depot antipsychotic injections should not be given at the same time as antipsychotic pills and syrups, but they often are. Care should be taken to establish the lowest possible dose to control the patient's symptoms, but often it is not. The side effects of depot antipsychotic injections are often more frequent and more severe than those of antipsychotic pills. Many patients are given high doses of depot antipsychotics over long periods of time without any review of their needs, thereby exposing them to increased risks of tardive dyskinesia, which is a consequence of the brain damage done by these drugs. According to a video produced by the Newcastle Medical School, 40 per cent of long-term psychiatric patients suffer from tardive dyskinesia.

People receiving treatment with depot antipsychotics should do all they can to get their medication reviewed regularly, but many will be unable to do so, either because they are so sedated by the drugs that they are effectively disabled, or because nobody would listen to them if they did ask for such a review. There is a growing body of evidence which points towards the possibility that high doses of antipsychotics taken over long periods of time may cause a supersensitivity in parts of the brain, causing people to become psychotic when they reduce the dose or stop taking the drugs. Some people call this condition tardive psychosis.

Studies looking into the effect of withdrawing antipsychotics from patients diagnosed as suffering from schizophrenia indicate that such patients are more likely to suffer a relapse than those who remain on maintenance doses of antipsychotics. Those who question the methods and interpretation of such studies are seen by the mainsteam of psychiatric opinion as heretics if they are psychiatrists, and dangerously naïve if they are not. The sceptical layperson will be aware that the economic weight and influence of the pharmaceutical industry is likely to balance the scales of research priorities in favour of finding medical, that is, pharmaceutical, solutions for the problems of living. That same sceptic will be equally aware that the drug industry spends vast sums of money to engage the best marketing brains to promote its wares as solutions. Social workers, psychologists, counsellors, psychotherapists and advocates are as relevant to the needs of people suffering from mental illness as drugs are, but they are all junior to the holder of the prescription pad.

Antipsychotic depot drugs have an almost unique potential for abuse. They can relieve the torment of terrifying symptoms of serious mental illness for many people, but they can also reduce a patient to an unprotesting zombie-like state. For some patients the best that depot antipsychotics will achieve for them will be the exchange of one form of human misery for another. Drowsiness, lethargy, loss of motivation, impotence, stiffened muscles, shaking hands, an inability to sit or stand still and persistent constipation may be more distressing to some people than a fixed belief that their thoughts are being controlled by the international brotherhood of Freemasons. For other people, of course, even side effects as serious as these may be a small price to pay for the relief that antipsychotic drugs give from a much more terrifying psychotic inner reality.

Starting on a course of antipsychotic depot injections is a major watershed in the life of an individual. For many it may be the start of a lifetime career as a mental patient attending a depot clinic for injections and a day centre to pack pencils into boxes for cigarette money. Getting the antipsychotic dose right for a particular patient can be difficult. It is very much easier to prescribe these powerful drugs in high doses which make the patient less demanding and more manageable. The quality of the services provided in Britain's mental hospitals and depot clinics varies enormously. The research team of Johnson and

Wright (1990) which looked at the prescribing practices in depot injection clinics stressed the need for 'constant vigilance in supervising the depot injection clinics.'

Five-Point Guide to Getting the Most from Antipsychotic Depot Injections

★ Antipsychotic depot drugs should not be routinely prescribed but used only when oral drugs have been shown to be inappropriate to the needs of the individual patient.

★ Anitpsychotic depot drugs should be prescribed in the lowest possible dose that meets the medical and social needs of the patient.

★ When depot antipsychotics are prescribed all other antipsychotics should be stopped.

★ The doses of depot antipsychotic drugs should be regularly reviewed with the patient and adjusted to the minimum required in the circumstances.

★ Depot antipsychotics should not be used to treat children or confused elderly people, patients under the influence of alcohol or other drugs which have a depressant action on the central nervous system, patients who suffer from Parkinsonism, or any patient with a known sensitivity to antipsychotic drugs.

FLUPENTHIXOL DECANOATE
(trade name Depixol)

General Information

Flupenthixol decanoate is used in the maintenance control of the symptoms of schizophrenia and other psychotic conditions. It is given by deep intramuscular injection into the buttock, which may be painful and cause swelling and small lumps at the site of the injection. The injection may be given once a fortnight or once a month.

Dosage Information

Adult (16 and over): A trial dose of 20 mg should be given to assess the patient's response to the drug before the treatment is started. If the drug causes the patient no serious adverse reactions, the treatment should begin five to ten days after the test dose with a further dose of between 20–40 mg, repeated at intervals of two to four weeks. The dose may be lowered or increased depending on the response of the patient. **The maximum dose is 400 mg per week**. The usual maintenance dosage range is from 50 mg every four weeks to 300 mg every two weeks. The progress of the patient should be very closely reviewed with a view to reducing the dose as soon as is practically possible.

Elderly and physically frail: Elderly people should start treatment with a quarter of the normal starting dose. Elderly and physically frail people are more prone to suffering from distressing side effects.

Children: Not recommended for the treatment of children.

Side Effects and Further Information

Flupenthixol may have a mood-lifting or alerting effect and so may be more helpful to depressed and withdrawn patients; it may cause violent or aggressive behaviour in agitated patients. If such a response occurs it may be necessary to change to another antipsychotic compound. The side effects of the drug occur within one to five days of the injection and reduce in severity after about five days. The side effects include lethargy, loss of motivation, muscular rigidity, tremors, physical restlessness, blurred vision, dry mouth and a mask-like facial expression. Where necessary these side effects may be reduced by other medications (for details of medications for side effects, see p. 165–9). Prolonged use may cause tardive dyskinesia, a condition which causes involuntary movements of the mouth, face, shoulders, trunk and limbs (for a fuller description of tardive dyskinesia see pp. 160–2).

FLUPHENAZINE DECANOATE

(trade name Modecate)

General Information

Fluphenazine decanoate used in the maintenance control of the symptoms of schizophrenia and other psychotic conditions. It is administered by deep intramuscular injection into the buttock. The injection may be given at regular intervals of between 14 and 35 days.

Dosage Information

Adult (16 and over): Before the treatment is started a trial dose of 12.5 mg should be given to assess the patient's response to the drug. If the drug is well tolerated, after an interval of between four and seven days a dose of between 12.5–100 mg may be given and repeated at intervals of 14 to 35 days. The dose may be adjusted upwards or downwards according to the response of the patient. As can be seen, the dose range of this drug is very wide, with the highest recommended dose eight times that of the lowest. The progress of patients should be very closely reviewed, with a view to reducing the dose as soon as is practically possible.

Elderly and physically frail: Elderly people should receive a trial dose of 6.25 mg (half the usual trial dose) and be treated with lower doses. Elderly and physically frail people are more prone to suffering from distressing side effects.

Children: Not recommended for the treatment of children.

Side Effects and Further Information

Fluphenazine should not be prescribed to patients who are severely depressed as it may seriously worsen the depression. It may take some days for the antipsychotic action of fluphenazine to take effect. Within hours of the injection extrapyramidal side effects may be experienced, such as a mask-like facial appearance, stiffening of limbs, inability to sit or stand still, blurred vision and loss of motivation. Prolonged use may cause tardive dyskinesia, a condition which causes involuntary movements of the mouth, face, shoulders, trunk and limbs (for a fuller description of tardive dykinesia see pp. 160–2). Where necessary these side effects may be reduced by other medications (for details of medications for side effects, see pp. 165-9.

FLUPHENAZINE ENANTHATE
(trade name Moditen)

General Information

Fluphenazine enanthate is for the maintenance control of schizophrenia and other psychotic conditions. It is very similar in its actions to fluphenazine decanoate (see previous entry), but its actions do not last as long and it causes extrapyramidal side effects more frequently than fluphenazine decanoate. It is administered by deep intramuscular injection into the buttock, which may be painful and cause swelling and small lumps at the site of the injection.

Dosage Information

Adult (16 and over): Before the treatment begins a trial dose of 12.5 mg should be given to test the patient's response to the drug. If the drug is well tolerated, after an interval of between four and seven days a dose of between 12.5–100 mg may be given and repeated at intervals of between 10 and 21 days. The dose may be increased or decreased according to the response of the patient.

Elderly and physically frail: Lower starting and maintenance doses should be used. Elderly and physically frail people are more prone to suffering from distressing side effects:

Children: Not recommended for the treatment of children.

Side Effects and Further Information

See the previous entry on fluphenazine decanoate.

FLUSPIRILINE
(trade name Redeptin)

General Information

Fluspiriline is used for the control of the symptoms of schizophrenia and other psychotic states. It is administered by deep intramuscular injection into the buttock, which may be painful and cause swelling and small lumps at the site of the injection. Fluspiriline is said to be less sedating than chlorpromazine and its side effects are said to compare favourably with other antipsychotic drugs used in similar doses.

Dosage Information

Adult (16 and over): Treatment begins with 2 mg per week, which may be increased in weekly increases of 2 mg until the desired response has been achieved. The usual maintenance dose is between 2–8 mg and **the maximum dose is 20 mg per week**. The progress of patients should be very closely reviewed, with a view to reducing the dose as soon as is practically possible.

Elderly and physically frail: Elderly people should begin treatment with a quarter to half the normal dose. Elderly and physically frail people are more prone to suffering from distressing side effects.

Children: Not recommended for the treatment of children.

Side Effects and Further Information

It may take some weeks before psychotic symptoms are relieved by fluspiriline. Common side effects are restlessness and sweating. Prolonged use may cause tardive dyskinesia, a condition which causes involuntary movements of the mouth, face, shoulders, trunk and limbs (for a fuller description of tardive dyskinesia see pp. 160–2). Where necessary these side effects may be reduced by other medications (for details of medications for side effects, see pp. 165–9).

HALOPERIDOL DECANOATE

(trade name Haldol)

General Information

Haloperidol decanoate is used for the maintenance control of schizophrenia and other psychotic conditions. It is administered by deep intramuscular injection into the buttock, which may be painful and cause swelling and small lumps at the site of the injection. It is less sedating than chlorpromazine but its other side effects may be more severe and more frequent.

Dosage Information

Adult (16 and over): Treatment begins with 50 mg every four weeks which if necessary may be increased after two weeks in steps of 50 mg to the usual **maximum dose of 300 mg every four weeks**. A small number of patients may be given higher doses. The progress of patients should be very closely reviewed, with a view to reducing the dose as soon as is practically possible.

Elderly and physically frail: Treatment begins with low doses (12.5 mg). Elderly and physically frail people are more prone to suffering from distressing side effects.

Children: Not recommended for the treatment of children.

Side Effects and Further Information

Haloperidol is less sedating than chlorpromazine but is more likely to cause extrapyramidal side effects such as inner agitation, physical restlessness, a mask-like facial appearance, tremors and muscular rigidity. Prolonged use may cause tardive dyskinesia, a condition which causes facial tics and other involuntary movements of the shoulders, trunk and limbs (for a fuller description of tardive dyskinesia, see pp. 160–2). Where necessary these side effects may be reduced by other medications (for details of medications for side effects, see pp. 165–9).

PIPOTHIAZINE PALMITATE
(trade name Piportil Depot)

General Information

Pipothiazine is used for the maintenance control of schizophrenia and other psychotic conditions. It is administered by deep intramuscular injection into the buttocks, which may be painful and cause swelling and small lumps at the site of the injection. Pipothiazine is said to have a moderately sedative action compared with chlorpromazine, to which it is related. This drug should be avoided in depressed patients as it may make the depression more severe.

Dosage Information

Adult (16 and over): Before treatment begins a trial dose of 25 mg should be given to test the patient's reaction to the drug. If the drug is well tolerated, after an interval of between four and seven days a dose of between 25–50 mg may be given and repeated at intervals of four weeks. The dose may be increased or decreased according to the response of the patient. The progress of patients should be very closely reviewed, with a view to reducing the dose as soon as is practically possible.

Elderly and physically frail: Treatment begins with 12.5 mg (half the usual starting dose). Elderly and physically frail people are more prone to suffering from distresing side effects.

Children: Not recommended for the treatment of children.

Side Effects and Further Information

Pipothiazine may cause severe Parkinsonism, a slowing of movements, stiffened arms, tremors, an expressionless facial appearance and some people's fingers may make a 'pill-rolling' movement. Prolonged use may cause tardive dyskinesia, a condition which causes involuntary movements of the mouth, face, shoulders, trunk and limbs (for a fuller description of tardive dyskinesia see pp. 160–2). Where necessary these side effects may be reduced by other medications (for details of medications for side effects, see pp. 165–9).

ZUCLOPENTHIXOL DECANOATE

(trade name Clopixol)

General Information

Zuclopenthixol decanoate is used for the maintenance control of schizophrenia and other psychotic conditions. It is administered by deep intramuscular injection into the buttocks, which may be painful and cause swelling and small lumps at the site of the injection. Zuclopenthixol should be avoided in porphyria, a rare inherited disorder caused by a disturbance in the way the body deals with the breakdown products of red blood cells. The disorder may be in the bone marrow, the liver or in both. The symptoms of porphyria are: sensitivity to sunlight, causing inflammation and blisters; inflammation of the nerves; mental disturbances; and attacks of abdominal pain. A form of porphyria is also associated with chronic alcoholism.

Dosage Information

Adult (16 and over): Before treatment begins a trial dose of 100 mg should be given to test the patient's reaction to the drug. If the drug is well tolerated, after an interval of between 7 and 28 days a dose of 100–200 mg or more may be given, followed at intervals of two to four weeks by doses of 200–400 mg. **The maximum dose is 600 mg per week**. The dose may be increased or decreased according to the response of the patient. The progress of patients should be very closely reviewed, with a view to reducing the dose as soon as is practically possible.

Elderly and physically frail: It is recommended that elderly people should be treated with one-fifth of the normal dose. Elderly and physically frail people are more prone to suffering from distressing side effects.

Children: Not recommended for the treatment of children.

Side Effects and Further Information

Zuoclopenthixol is said to be useful for the treatment of agitated or aggressive patients. It is said to be less sedating than chlorpromazine, to have fewer extrapyramidal side effects, but to cause more Parkinsonism-like side effects. Prolonged use may cause tardive dyskinesia, a condition which causes involuntary movements of the mouth, face, shoulders, trunk and limbs (for a fuller description of tardive dyskinesia and its side effects, see pp. 160–2).

Antipsychotic Drugs: Side Effects and Further Information

The following list of side effects applies to all the antipsychotic drugs listed in this guide. There are, however, differences between some of the drugs in the severity and frequency with which the side effects occur. Another complicating factor is that antipsychotic drugs affect different people in different ways and some people are much more likely than others to find side effects distressing. Elderly and physically frail people are much more vulnerable to serious side effects than those who are younger and fitter. Two other factors also affect the severity of the side effects:

The dose of the drug taken: The higher the dose, the more frequent and more severe will be the side effects. In higher doses antipsychotics are more likely to cause tardive dyskinesia (see below).

The number of drugs taken: The more different drugs taken, the more frequent and more severe will be the side effects. The combination of antidepressants with antipsychotics may mean that the side effects of both drugs are felt. Such combinations may also increase the risk of tardive dyskinesia as tricyclic antidepressants are very closely related to phenothiazine antipsychotics and have many similar effects. The medications given to relieve the side effects of antipsychotic drugs also increase the risk of tardive dyskinesia.

The best results for the patient are achieved when antipsychotic drugs are used at the lowest effective dose for the needs of individual patient and when they are used with as few other drugs as possible.

If you are troubled by side effects you should notify the prescribing doctor and, if necessary, not hesitate to make a nuisance of yourself until you are satisfied that the drugs and doses prescribed have been tailored to your own particular needs.

Side Effects – How Serious and How Common?

Antipsychotic drugs do not have exactly the same effects and side effects for everyone and many of them vary depending on the dose given. Some people will require higher doses to obtain relief from their symptoms than others, and some will suffer from the side effects of antipsychotic drugs more severely at lower doses than others. Elderly and physically frail people are much more prone than younger or physically fitter people to be caused distress by side effects. People taking antipsychotic drugs frequently become lethargic and lose motivation, and it is highly probable that they may not complain about side effects unless they are pressed to discuss them. However, whenever patients are asked generally about things which trouble them, the side effects of their drugs feature very prominently amongst their concerns. The experience of side effects is first and foremost a subjective experience which is extremely difficult, if not impossible, to measure scientifically with any degree of reliability. It is generally accepted that the adverse effects of prescribed drugs are under-reported. The prescribers' handbooks do give some broad indications as to the frequency of the side effects of individual drugs, but the reliability of such indications is suspect in so far as they imply a degree of sensitivity on the part of the prescribers which is not always evident in the reported prescribing practices of psychiatry. The purpose of this guide is not to reassure people about the effects of psychiatric drugs or to encourage them to take them, but to validate their experiences and empower them in informed discussions with their doctors. For these reasons the side effects listed below are not classified according to their frequency or their severity. Although it should be remembered that not everyone will experience or notice all of the side effects listed here, if a drug is being considered the possibility of side effects should enter into that consideration, and the worries of the person taking the drug should not be dismissed simply by telling him or her that a side effect is 'rare'. Unless otherwise stated, all the side effects listed below are only a problem whilst the drugs are being taken.

Eyes: Blurred vision. Miosis (narrowing of the pupil). Perphenazine and trifluoperazine can cause mydraisis (widening of the pupil). With long-term use, the pigmentation of the retina, conjunctiva and cornea of the eye, which may impair vision.

Stomach and bladder: Constipation. Decreased secretion of gastric fluids and reduced reflex movements of the stomach. Decreased saliva (dry mouth). Nausea. Rarely, reduced urination.

Sexual functions: Reduced sexual arousal. Difficulty in achieving orgasm. Impotence. Sterility. Menstrual periods may become irregular or stop. Galactorrhoea (the production of milk in the breasts). Rarely, gynaecomastia (abnormal enlargement of the breasts in men). Reduction in the size and weight of testicles.

Body temperature regulation: Patients on antipsychotics are more vulnerable to hypothermia (reduced body temperature) in cold weather and hyperthermia (increased body temperature) in hot weather.

Brain: 'Pseudo-Parkinsonism', which can cause a mask-like facial expression, muscular rigidity, shaking hands, disturbed balance, stiffening of the neck, a shuffling walk (often referred to in England as the 'Modecate' or 'Largactil shuffle' and in the US the 'Prolixin stomp'), apathy and depression. Approximately one-third of patients treated with normal doses of antipsychotic drugs will be affected by pseudo-Parkinsonism. Reduced seizure threshold, increasing the risk of epileptic fits in people prone to suffering them. When high doses are used, there is a risk that people with no previous history of or disposition to epileptic seizures may suffer fits. Nightmares. Insomnia. Akathisia (inner agitation and restlessness, anxiety and an inability to sit or stand still). Tardive dyskinesia (see p. 160), a condition which appears to be permanent in some patients. Long-term use may cause dopamine receptor (nerve cells in the brain involved in the transmission of messages) supersensitivity, which may cause a worsening of the symptoms of schizophrenia when antipsychotic drugs are withdrawn.

Skin: Photosensitivity (increased risk of sunburn after moderate exposure). Pallor. Sweating. With long-term use, purplish pigmentation of the skin. Rashes. One in twenty patients may expect to suffer skin problems. With injected antipsychotics, small nodules may appear at the site of the injections. Jaundice (see below), which causes a characteristic yellow skin tint.

Liver: Obstructive jaundice (a form of jaundice caused by the obstruction of bile ducts).

Autoimmune system: Very rarely, a condition resembling lupus erythematosus, a disease which affects the skin and internal organs. The most common sign is a red scaly rash on the face, affecting the nose and cheeks, arthritis and progressive damage to the kidney. In its mildest forms only the skin is affected. It can render patients more prone to catching infections.

Heart, circulation and blood: Reduced blood pressure which can cause the patient to feel faint when standing. Occasionally patients may faint. Changes in rate of heart beat. Pimozide has been associated with sudden deaths, which are caused by its effects on the heart (see p. 123). Agranulocytosis (a condition in which damage to the bone marrow causes a serious deficiency of white blood cells). Although this condition is very rare (it is estimated that 1 in 10,000 patients will suffer it), it may lead rapidly to collapse and death. Another rare side effect is haemolytic anaemia (the destruction of red blood cells).

Body weight: Weight gain, which can be substantial.

The neuroleptic malignant syndrome: The neuroleptic malignant syndrome (NMS) is a rare and potentially fatal side effect of antipsychotic drugs whose exact cause is unknown. Of patients who are affected by NMS approximately one in five die. Studies into the frequency of NMS put the risk between two and ten patients per thousand, but these figures may be an overestimate. The symptoms of NMS include changing states of consciousness, rapidly increased body temperature, muscular rigidity, pale skin, increased heart rate, urinary incontinence, changes in breathing and sweating. There is no treatment which has been proved to be effective for NMS. The condition appears to last for as long as the antipsychotic drug remains in the body; for between five and ten days with tablets, syrup, or short-term injections, but two weeks or longer with depot preparations.

Tardive dyskinesia: Translated from the Latin, tardive dyskinesia means involuntary movement of late onset and constitutes the most common and most worrying hazard associated with the use of antipsychotic drugs. The symptoms of TD are:

Facial movments. A constant sucking of the lips. Movements of the jaw from side to side with the mouth partially open. darting, 'fly-catching' and rolling movements of the tongue. Frowning or raising of the eyebrows. Grimacing. Increased blinking and rolling of the eyes.

Movements of the neck and shoulders. A rolling motion of the neck and a persistent, slow rolling and shrugging movement of the shoulders.

Movements of the limbs. Spreading, twisting and 'piano-playing' movements of the fingers. Spreading movements of the toes. Foot tapping and a rotating movement of the ankles.

Movements of the trunk. Pelvic thrusting movement.

Breathing and swallowing movements. Disturbances in breathing rhythm which may be accompanied by animal-like grunting noises. Swallowing may be difficult.

These movements are beyond the person's control and tend to disappear whilst he or she is alseep. They are usually first noticed when antipsychotic drugs are reduced in dose or withdrawn. The only effective way to control them is by administering more of the drug which caused them in the first place and thus exposing the patient to the risk of making the underlying condition worse. In its most severe and extremely rare form, TD can be a crippling condition.

A small minority of psychiatrists do not accept that TD is caused by antipsychotic drugs. They point to the fact that Emil Kraepelin, the psychiatrist who first classified the group of symptoms which we now call schizophrenia, described involuntary movements similar to those of TD in his patients at the beginning of the century, long before the discovery of chlorpromazine, the first antipsychotic drug. However, the main body of opinion is that TD is a condition which is caused by the use of antipsychotic drugs, usually after years of use of the drugs and very rarely after a single dose.

It is very difficult to predict the statistical risk of contracting TD: estimates of its prevalence vary from just over 5 per cent of people receiving long-term treatment with antipsychotic drugs to as high as 56 per cent. This wide discrepancy arises because different researchers have used different criteria to define TD. The most widely accepted figure for the number of people who are treated with antipsychotics for periods of three years or longer and who develop TD is 20 per cent, or one in five. The risk of TD is thought to be highest for elderly patients and in particular for elderly female patients. Women patients tend to be treated with higher doses of antipsychotic drugs than men, so this increased risk of TD may well be a reflection of this factor, rather than of any gender-related biological differences between men and women. Although the elderly do seem to be at more risk of suffering TD, it is reported in younger patients, including adolescents. Another major risk factor in

TD is the dose of antipsychotics taken, the higher the dose the greater the risk of being affected. The use of drugs to treat the side effects of antipsychotic drugs may also increase the risk of TD.

TD has been described in medical literature as a 'major public health hazard' and 'probably the most commonly diagnosed iatrogenic [a condition caused by treatment] disorder of the central nervous system.' A training video called 'Tardive Dyskinesia Observed', produced for doctors by the Newcastle Medical School, estimates that 40 per cent of all chronic (long-term) patients treated with antipsychotics have TD to some degree. It has increasingly come to be regarded as the stigmata of the modern psychiatric patient, marking him or her out in the community.

Tardive dyskinesia can seriously diminish a person's quality of life, also his or her prospects of resuming a valued role in the community. The short-term side effects of antipsychotic drugs alone are sufficiently serious to require the greatest degree of care in the way they are prescribed and used and the risk that patients may be disfigured by the strange movements and tics caused by TD adds to the urgency of the need to improve the quality of prescribing practices in psychiatry. As a number of people diagnosed as schizophrenic will not suffer a relapse for many years, if at all, after their first episode, this raises the issue as to whether such patients and their relatives should be offered a trial of drug-free management of the symptoms and the resulting stresses. The combination of side effects and TD leads to the conclusion that antipsychotic drugs should only be used for the treatment of very serious mental illness.

How antipsychotics interact with other drugs and medicines	
Drug	*Result of interaction*
Alcohol	Increased drowsiness.
Anaesthetics	Increased reduction of blood pressure.
Indomethacin painkillers such as *Flexus Continus; *Indocid & Indocid R, *Indocid PDA, *Indolar SR, *Indomod, *Rheumacin, *Slo-Indo	Severe drowsiness when given with haloperidol.

Antacids	Reduced absorption of phenothiazines.
Rifampicin antibacterial drugs such as *Rifadin, *Rifatar, *Rifinah 150 and 300, *Rimactane, *Rimactazid 150 and 300	Haloperidol is metabolized more quickly, which reduces the amount of haloperidol in the blood, thereby reducing its effects.
Tricyclic antidepressants	Increased side effects of phenothiazines.
MAOI antidepressants	Increased blood pressure and excitation with oxypertin (*Integrin).
Anti-epileptics	Antipsychotics reduce the effectiveness of anti-epileptic drugs. Carbamazepine (*Tegretol, *Tegretol Retard) increases the rate at which haloperidol is metabolized.
Drugs used to reduce blood pressure	Increased reduction of blood pressure. Increased risk of extrapyramidal side effects with methyldopa (*Aldomet, *Dopamet), metirosine (*Demser) and reserpine (*Decaserpil, *Hypercal, *Serpasil).
Antimuscarinic drugs, for example drugs used to treat bronchitis, such as *Atrovent, *Rinatec. **Drugs used to treat side effects of antipsychotics such as *Artane, *Cogentin, *Disipal, *Kemedrin.** **Also similar drugs used in the treatment of bladder and stomach disorders.**	Reduces the concentration of phenothiazine antipsychotics. May increase the likelihood of tardive dyskinesia. Increased extrapyramidal side effects. If the patient has tardive dyskinesia this will be 'unmasked'. See discussion of medicines for side effects on pp. 165–9.
Tranquillizers and sleeping pills.	Increased drowsiness and sedation.
	* = TRADE NAME

Conditions in which Antipsychotic Drugs Must be Avoided

Comatose patients. Bone marrow deficiencies. Glaucoma (a
condition in which pressure in the eye is abnormally high). See
also the listings for individual drugs.

**Conditions in which Antipsychotic Drugs Should be Used
with Caution**

Old age (70 and over). Heart disease. Diseases of the blood
vessels in the brain. Respiratory diseases (pneumonia, pleurisy,
etc.). Phaeochromocytoma (a tumour in the adrenal gland
which causes increased blood pressure and heart rate, palpitations and headaches). Parkinsonism. Epilepsy. Serious infections. Pregnancy. Breast-feeding. Liver disease. Kidney disease.
History of jaundice. Leucopenia (a reduction in the white blood
cells). Hypothyroidism (a reduced function of the thyroid gland,
causing reduced metabolism, tiredness and lethargy). Myasthe-
nia gravis (a chronic disease marked by severe fatigue and
muscular weakness which can cause temporary paralysis).
Enlarged prostate gland (most common in elderly men). Caution should be exercised in elderly or frail people in very hot or
cold weather. Patients given intramuscular injections should
remain lying down for 30 minutes after receiving the injection.

Drugs for the Treatment of the Side Effects of Antipsychotics (Anti-Parkinsonian Drugs)

As this guide shows, all antipsychotic drugs have a wide range
of serious, unwanted effects which are often sufficiently
distressing to warrant treatment in their own right, and
amongst these 'pseudo-Parkinsonism' may be the most troublesome. The drugs used to treat these side effects are the same as
the drugs used to treat Parkinsonism and are referred to as
anticholinergics or antimuscularinics, but for the sake of
simplicity and clarity the term used in this guide is anti-
Parkinsonian drugs. These drugs have their own unwanted
effects and problems associated with their use, and although
they can reduce some of the side effects of antipsychotics, they
do so at a price. That price is the exchange of one set of

unwanted effects for another, hopefully more tolerable, set of side effects and an increased exposure to the risk of tardive dyskinesia. High doses of antipsychotics increase the severity and frequency of their side effects. Patients on high doses are therefore more likely to be given medication for the control of side effects, and as a consequence they are also at greater risk of suffering permanent damage to their central nervous system. Antipsychotic drugs can actually mask Tardive dyskinesia, but it is usually revealed when the dose of antipsychotic is reduced or the drug stopped. It may also be revealed by anti-Parkinsonian medication.

Anti-Parkinsonian drugs are often routinely administered with antipsychotic drugs, which is extremely controversial. The World Health Organization recently issued a consensus statement on the use of anti-Parkinsonian drugs in which the arguments against their routine use was summarized as follows: '(a) The long-term use of anticholinergics may predispose to tardive dyskinesia (in fact, the administration of these agents exacerbates the syndrome in affected patients and has been used as an aid to its early detection). (b) Anticholinergic medication may induce autonomic side effects, which may be sometimes serious (urinary retention, paralytic ileus). (c) The long-term use of anticholinergics is likely to affect memory functions, and thus further compromise the already impaired cognitive performance of schizophrenic patients. (d) It has been suggested that anticholinergics may contribute to the development of hyperthermic episodes, some of which may be fatal. (e) The consumption of an excessive dose of anticholinergics may produce an acute toxic state, with agitation, disorientation in time and space, delusions and hallucinations. (f) In some cases, anticholinergics may be abused as euphoriants, so that their discontinuation may be difficult. (g) There are some indications that anticholinergics can decrease the therapeutic activity of neuroleptics, although early reports of pharmacokinetic interactions between the two classes of drugs have not been confirmed by more recent studies. (h) Many patients on antipsychotic therapy do not develop Parkinsonism, so that preventative treatment is sometimes useless.'

The WHO consensus statement concludes: 'On the basis of these considerations, the propylactic use of anticholinergics in patients on neuroleptic treatment is not recommended, and may be justified only early in treatment (after which it should be discontinued and its need should be re-evaluated). As a rule these compounds should only be used when Parkinsonism has actually developed, and when other measures, such as the reduction of neuroleptic dosage or the substitution of the administered drug by another less prone to induce Parkinsonism, have proven ineffective.'

The following is a list and description of Anti-Parkinsonian drugs.

BENZHEXOL

Trade name	Description
Artane	2 mg white tablets marked Lederle 4434. 5 mg white tablets marked Lederle 4436.
Bentex	2 mg white tablets. 5 mg white tablets.
Broflex	Pink syrup for dilution to be taken orally.
Benzhexol (generic name)	2 mg white tablets. 5 mg white tablets.

General Information

Benzhexol is used for the treatment of Parkinsonism and the side effects of antipsychotic drugs. It may have a stimulating effect.

Dosage Information

Treatment begins with 1 mg (half a tablet) per day, taken before or after meals, and gradually increased to the usual maintenance dose of between 5–15 mg per day in three to four divided doses.

BENZTROPINE	
Trade name	*Description*
Cogentin	2 mg white tablets marked MSD 60. Injection (for emergency treatment of very severe side effects of antipsychotics).

General Information

Benztropine is used for the treatment of Parkinsonism and the side effects of antipsychotic drugs. It causes drowsiness or sedation rather than stimulation.

Dosage Information

By mouth: Treatment begins with between 0.5–1 mg per day, taken at bedtime and gradually increased to **a maximum dose of 6 mg per day**. The usual maintenance dose is 1–4 mg per day.

By injection: 1–2 mg repeated if symptoms reappear.

ORPHENADRINE	
Trade name	*Description*
Biorphen	Liquid to be taken orally.
Disipal	50 mg yellow tablets marked Disipal.

General Information

Orphenadrine is used for the treatment of Parkinsonism and the side effects of antipsychotic drugs. It may cause more stimulation and euphoria than benzhexol. It should be avoided in porphyria, a rare inherited disorder caused by a disturbance in the way in which the body deals with the breakdown products of red blood cells. The disorder may be in the bone marrow, the liver or both. The symptoms of porphyria are sensitivity to sunlight, which causes inflammation and blisters, inflammation of the nerves, mental disturbances and attacks of abdominal pain. A form of porphyria is also associated with chronic alcoholism.

Dosage Information

Treatment begins with 150 mg per day in divided doses, increased gradually to **a maximum dose of 400 mg per day**.

PROCYCLIDINE	
Trade name	*Description*
Kemadrin	5 mg white tablets. Injection (for emergency treatment of very severe side effects of antipsychotics).
Arpicolin	Syrup to be taken orally.
Procyclidine (generic name)	5 mg white tablets.

General Information

Procyclidine is used for the treatment of Parkinsonism and the side effects of antipsychotic drugs. It may have a stimulating effect.

Dosage Information

By mouth: Treatment begins with 2.5–3 mg per day, increased if necessary to **a maximum dose of 30 mg per day, or up to 60 mg per day in rare circumstances**.

By intramuscular injection: For immediate treatment of very severe side effects, 5–10 mg, repeated if necessary after 20 minutes. **The maximum dose is 20 mg per day**.

By intramuscular injection: For maintenance treatment 5 mg; rarely 10 mg or more.

Anti-Parkinsonian Drugs: Side Effects and Further Information

The drugs listed in this section are almost identical in their actions but some tend to stimulate whilst others sedate (this information is given for each product under its heading above). These drugs should not be suddenly stopped but should be withdrawn gradually. Some patients have hoarded these drugs and taken them in high doses in order to get 'high' and one researcher has suggested that in such circumstances the patients might be doing this as a form of self-medication in order to counter the depressing and mood-flattening effects of antipsychotic drugs.

Side Effects

Dry mouth. Stomach upsets. Dizziness. Blurred vision.

Less Common Side Effects

Changes in heart rhythm. Hypersensitivity (an abnormally high sensitivity to the drugs which results in the patient having allergic-type reactions to them). With high doses some patients may experience confusion, excitement, and psychotic reactions; in these circumstances the drug should be withdrawn.

Conditions in which Anti-Parkinsonian Drugs Should Be Used with Caution

Difficulty with urination. Glaucoma (a condition in which the pressure inside the eye is abnormally high). Heart and blood circulation disease. Liver disease. Kidney disease.

Introduction

Manic depression is characterized by moods which swing dramatically between the depths of depression and euphoric 'highs'. It can appear without warning, and occasionally it vanishes just as mysteriously. In the depressed phase of the illness the sufferer sinks to the lowest despair and in the manic phase is driven by euphoric flights of fantasy. Between periods of deep depression and mania the individual will lead a perfectly ordinary and unremarkable life. Many sufferers are creative and successful people, but many more live on a razor's edge of potential disaster. In the depressive phase the sufferer may be suicidal, but in the manic phase he or she may be abnormally and destructively sexually promiscuous, prone to making disastrous financial decisions driven by unshakeable belief in a fantasised opportunity. Antipsychotic drugs are often used to bring people down from their psychotic highs, with antidepressants used to treat their depression. Lithium is used to stabilize and prevent these mood swings and for about 70 per cent of people who suffer from manic depression it is very successful.

The lightest of all metals, lithium is a naturally occurring element which was discovered in 1817. It has been used to treat a wide variety of conditions. In the middle of the last century it was used as a treatment for gout, in the 1920s as a sleeping draft and in the 1940s as a sodium substitute. This therapeutic pragmatism with Lithium had disastrous and frequently fatal consequences. Lithium was first tried as a treatment for manic depression in 1949 by an Australian called Cade. In the course of some experiments, Cade noticed that guinea pigs became lethargic when injected with lithium. From this observation he took a mighty leap in the dark and gave it to some manic depressive patients. In 1949 he published a paper showing that in ten out of ten patients lithium had achieved positive results. However, at that time there was little interest in the psychiatric community in Cade's findings. Lithium's track record in medicine had until then been punctuated by a succession of lethal disasters, and psychiatry was about to embark on its honeymoon with chlorpromazine, the first of the antipsychotics. The fact that lithium was a naturally occurring element beyond the scope of patenting possibilities also meant that it did not have much appeal to the pharmaceutical industry. Cade's discovery did not, therefore, attract the marketing razzmatazz usual in the world of the hospitality-addicted prescribers. It was not until 1968, when a Danish psychiatrist called Schou reported positive findings in the prevention of both depressive and manic phases of the illness, that lithium began to gain respectability as a treatment.

Just how lithium exerts its effects on manic depression remains a matter of theory and speculation, and its precise actions remain as mysterious as those of other psychiatric drugs. It is one of the most toxic substances used in medicine and the line between its therapeutic and toxic doses is very narrow indeed. For this reason considerable care is needed in establishing the correct dose for the individual. Given the extreme distress which manic depression can cause the sufferer and those around him or her, the side effects of lithium are usually rather minor, but they can be hazardous to some people.

LITHIUM CARBONATE

Trade name	Description
Camcolit 250 **Camcolit 400**	250 mg white tablets marked Camcolit. 400 mg white tablets marked Camcolit S.
Liskonum	450 mg white tablets.
Phasal	300 mg white tablets marked P.
Priadel	200 mg white tablets marked P200. 400 mg white tablets marked PRIADEL.

LITHIUM CITRATE

Trade name	Description
Litarex	564 mg white tablets.

General Information

Lithium is used to stabilize the moods of people suffering from manic depression and to prevent both the depressive lows and manic peaks. It is not a cure for the illness, but it does help many sufferers to lead productive and enjoyable lives by controlling at least the worst of the symptoms. Lithium does not work for all patients, neither does it affect all patients uniformly. Whilst taking lithium care must be taken to ensure an adequate fluid and salt intake. Patients should drink at least four to six pints of liquid a day, but use alcohol in moderation because it can cause bodily fluid loss. It is also wise to take at least an average amount of salt with food. Hot weather and heavy work which causes sweating can be hazardous when on lithium. At the outset of treatment it is necessary to have the efficiency of kidneys and thyroid glands checked. Before maintenance treatment is begun the dose level for the particular patient has to be established. This is done by testing the serum level (the concentration of lithium in the blood) of lithium on the fourth and seventh days of treatment, and thereafter every seven days until the appropriate dose level has been established and stabilized. It may take a number of attempts before the correct dose for an individual patient is established. Blood tests should be repeated monthly until the dose has been stabilized for some time, after which they may be given at slightly longer intervals. These tests are vitally important, not only to prevent damage to the patient's health from too high levels of lithium, but also to reduce the risk of a relapse should the level get too low.

Dosage Information

Adult (16 and over): *Lithium carbonate*: Treatment begins with 0.25–2 g per day, adjusted to the level appropriate for the individual patient.

Lithium citrate: Treatment begins with 564 mg twice daily, adjusted to the level appropriate for the individual patient.

Elderly and physically frail: Elderly and physically frail people should receive reduced dosage.

Children: Lithium is not suitable for the treatment of children.

OVERDOSE EXTREMELY DANGEROUS · SEEK IMMEDIATE MEDICAL HELP

Side Effects and Further Information

Early side effects are: Increased thirst. Increased urination. Nausea. Mild stomach upsets. Trembling hands. Slight muscular weakness. Dry mouth. Decreased interest in sex. Slight dizziness. Aggravated acne.

Intermediate side effects are: Excessive weight gain. Excessive urination. Skin rash. Kidney damage. Damage to the thyroid gland, causing tiredness, slowing of mental processes, dry skin, aching muscles, feelings of cold and trembling hands.

Serious side effects are: Persistent diarrhoea. Severe nausea and vomiting. Severe hand tremors. Frequent muscular twitching. Blurred vision. Confusion. Serious discomfort. Goitre (a benign swelling of the thyroid gland). These serious side effects could be caused by the level of lithium in the blood becoming dangerously high. Urgent medical attention must be sought.

Conditions in which Lithium Must be Avoided

Kidney disease. Heart disease. Addison's disease (a condition in which there is an inadequate secretion of certain hormones in the adrenal glands, causing weakness, loss of energy, low blood pressure and darkening of the skin).

Conditions in which Lithium Should be Used with Caution

Treatment with diuretics (which increase urination). The long-term use of lithium causes changes in the kidneys and to the thyroid gland. Therefore it is clear that lithium should be used only for severe manic depressive psychosis. It is recommended that the use of lithium should be very carefully reviewed after three to five years, with a view to stopping it. Caution is necessary in elderly and physically frail people, when reduced doses should be used.

Use in Pregnancy and Breast-feeding

Women who are not pregnant at the start of treatment with lithium may be offered contraceptive advice and counselling. If a woman becomes pregnant whilst taking lithium serious consideration may be given to stopping the lithium or substituting it with another less hazardous medication, such as an antipsychotic or an antidepressant. Lithium is hazardous to the unborn child. Breast-feeding is strongly advised against. Very sensitive judgements must be made in balancing the needs of the mother against those of the child.

CARBAMAZEPINE

Trade name	Description
Carbamazepine (generic)	100 mg white tablets. 200 mg white tablets. 400 mg white tablets.
Tegretol	100 mg white tablets marked TEGRETOL 100. 200 mg white tablets marked TEGRETOL 200. 400 mg white tablets marked GEIGY/GEIGY on one side TEGRETOL on the other.

General Information

Carbamazepine is most commonly used as a treatment for epilepsy but is also sometimes used in the treatment of manic depression for patients who do not have a good response to lithium.

Dosage Information

Treatment begins with 400 mg per day in divided doses which may be increased if necessary until the desired effect is achieved to a **maximum dose of 1600 mg per day**. Usual dose between 400–600 mg/per day.

Elderly and physically frail: Treatment begins with a lower starting dose and should be increased in smaller steps than for healthy adults.

Side Effects and Further Information

The side effects of carbamazepine are less likely to be distressing if the treatment is started by gradually increasing the dose until the desired effect of stabilizing the mood swings in manic depression have been achieved. They are also said to become less of a problem to the patient after about two weeks of treatment. A wide range of side effects have been reported in patients using carbamazepine but not all patients will experience all of these. Dizziness. Headache. Visual disturbances. In elderly patients confusion and agitation. Dry mouth. Nausea. Diarrhoea. Loss of appetite. Tiredness. Ataxia (unsteady walk, shaky movements and difficulty with speech.) Skin rashes (possibly three in every 100 patients). Regular blood tests are recommended as carbamazepine sometimes causes serious blood disorders.

Conditions in Which Carbamazepine Must be Avoided

People taking MAOI antidepressants. Atriventricular abnormalities (muscles in the heart which control rate of heartbeat).

Conditions in Which Carbamazepine Should be Used with Caution

Severe heart disease. Kidney disease. Liver disease.

Introduction

Central nervous system (CNS) stimulants are drugs which can cause feelings of excitement, tension, increased energy, euphoria and paranoia. The best-known CNS stimulants are amphetamines which are probably most well known for their reputation as recreational drugs and are often collectively referred to as 'uppers' or 'speed'. Amphetamines and similar drugs can cause dependence very rapidly and once hooked, regular users need to increase the doses they take in order to ward off the profound depression that comes when the level of the drug in their bodies falls. Nowadays CNS stimulants have very few uses in medicine. They have been used to treat depression, but this was abandoned when experience showed that not only were they ineffective, they often made people feel worse and gave them a drug problem in the process. Stimulants have also been promoted and prescribed as 'anorexiants' or appetite suppressants and the use of these drugs as slimming aids has led to many women becoming hooked on them, only to find themselves and their drug problems abandoned when CNS stimulants went out of fashion with the doctors who had previously prescribed them so freely.

CNS stimulants are now suggested for three purposes: to treat narcolepsy, to lift the moods of people suffering from 'institutionalism' or recovering from illness, and to make so-called 'hyperkinetic' (overactive) children more obedient and attentive. Narcolepsy is a very rare condition where sufferers have a powerful tendency to fall asleep in quiet surroundings or whilst engaged in monotonous activities. Institutionalism is a state of mind and being caused by long periods of living in depersonalizing institutions, of which the most extreme examples are mental hospitals and prisons. The individual adapts to the rhythms and demands of the institution to the extent that his or her capacity to act independently or cope outside the institution is seriously impaired. Often the institutionalized individual becomes apathetic, dependent on others and lacks any sense of cause and effect in his or her own behaviour. The problems of institutionalism can be all the more severe in mental hospitals, where patients spend years on end permanently and routinely sedated by powerful drugs. Mental-hospital staff often refer to their institutionalized patients as 'burnt-out schizophrenics', thus conveniently attributing their condition to the disease rather than to the treatment. The victims of institutionalism can be seen in the back wards of many mental hospitals with nicotine-stained fingers twitching as they watch children's television; in day centres performing mindless tasks euphemistically described as occupational therapy; and, increasingly, amongst the growing populations of cardboard cities around Britain. The manufacturers of Villescon™, a compound combining a mild stimulant with vitamins, include 'institutional neuroses' amongst the uses for their product.

All the stimulants listed in the British National Formulary are suggested as being potentially useful for the treatment of hyperkinesis in children. Whilst it is by no means controversial that some children are overactive, the medical labels given to this age-old and universal problem are very controversial indeed. Youngsters who might otherwise be described as bloody little nuisances can be transformed into medical problems by attaching impressive labels to their behaviour. Thus, Denis the Menace, Beryl the Peril and Just William might, if they lived in the real world, be diagnosed as suffering from 'Hyperkinetic Syndrome', 'Minimal Brain Dysfunction', 'Functional Behaviour Problems' or 'Hyperkinetic Impulse Disorder', and be prescribed drugs to make them better. All these 'diagnoses' are extremely broad and ill defined. Overactivity, short attention span, poor powers of concentration, low frustration tolerance, impulsive and explosive temperament – these have become 'symptoms' to be measured by child psychiatrists, teachers and parents. Once the diagnosis is made Denis, Beryl and William will be given amphetamines, which will have the paradoxical effect of making them more subdued, rather than stimulating them to commit further outrages to the sensibilities of their parents and teachers. The same effect might be achieved by giving them a snort of cocaine, also a CNS stimulant and no more or less dangerous a drug than those which might actually be prescribed.

Drugs such as amphetamines retard a child's growth and there is a lack of evidence as to whether this retarded growth is made up later in the child's life or is permanent. Studies of children treated with stimulants do not show that their long-term chances in life are enhanced by the treatment. The pharmaceutical industry has played a major part in promoting the diagnosis of hyperactivity syndrome. In the United States the pharmaceutical giant CIBA actively encouraged its salesmen to promote their product, Ritalin FBP (Functional Behaviour Problems), amongst teachers, social workers and probation officers and this early promotional activity was extremely influential. In 1973, Grinspoon and Singer, two workers at Harvard University, concluded in a scholarly review of the use of amphetamines amongst children in America that 'the possible adverse effects of these drugs and their unknown long-term risks require that we reconsider the present policy of amphetamines in the schools.'[7] Three years before they conducted their review, a spokesman for the Food and Drugs Administration was quoted as estimating that between 150,000 and 200,000 children were being treated with these drugs in America. At the same time, the National Institute of Mental Health was suggesting that there were up to four million children 'who could benefit from these drugs.' Amphetamine use never reached anything like this scale in Britain, but the issues raised by Grinspoon and Singer have still not been resolved and are still just as important, whether they apply to hundreds of children, or hundreds of thousands.

DEXAMPHETAMINE SULPHATE

Trade name	Description
Dexadrine	5 mg white tablets marked SK&F.

General Information

Dexamphetamine is a potent stimulant which is used in the treatment of narcolepsy and for the so-called hyperkinetic syndrome in children. It is the most powerful CNS stimulant in current use in the Health Service. Dexamphetamine is a widely abused drug because of its ability to produce feelings of energetic well-being, alertness and sociability. Tolerance to these effects develops very quickly, usually within two to three

[7]Grinspoon, L. and Singer, S. B.: 'Amphetamines in the Treatment of Hyperkinetic Children': *Harvard Educational Review*, 43, pp. 515–55, 1973.

weeks, which leads abusers to increase steadily the dose they take in order to ward off the feelings of agitated anxiety and profound depression which occur as the effects of the drug wear off. The high doses taken by habitual abusers often causes 'amphetamine psychosis', in which the user is tormented by paranoid fears and anxieties, delusions and hallucinations. An individual in this state is terrified by a fixed belief that he or she is being persecuted or punished, hears taunting voices, feels that insects are crawling under his or her skin, gnashes his or her teeth uncontrollably, and feels unremitting terror and rage. This state can be sufficiently severe to require admission to hospital. Not all people who use amphetamines recreationally necessarily reach this state; some users take the drug occasionally to enhance their social lives or their capacity to work. In such circumstances the greatest risk run by people who use amphetamines unlawfully is the risk of arrest and prosecution by the police.

Dosage Information

For the treatment of narcolepsy. 10 mg per day in divided doses, increased if necessary to **a maximum dose of 60 mg per day**.

Children: for the treatment of hyperactive children aged between three and five: 2.5 mg daily in the morning, increased if necessary by 2.5 mg per day at weekly intervals, to **a maximum dose of 20 mg per day**.

For hyperactive children aged between six and twelve: 5–10 mg per day in the morning, increased if necessary by 5 mg per day at weekly intervals, to **a maximum dose of 40 mg per day**.

This highly controversial treatment should only be given in circumstances where the social and psychological needs of the child and the family can be met in an effective and sensitive manner. In many parts of the country such services are either unavailable or inadequate, and in these circumstances there is no justification for using this method of dealing with the child's problems. The long-term outcome of this treatment is uncertain. There is an unmeasured risk that the child's physical growth may be permanently impaired. There is also the risk that the child may come to believe that drugs provide an easy solution to life's problems.

Side Effects and Further Information

There is a high risk of addiction to dexamphetamine. Whilst children are taking this drug their growth is impaired and it is not known whether or not this is a permanent effect. In the short-term a marked improvement in a child's behaviour may be observed, but this may be bought at an unjustifiable risk to the child. The side effects of dexamphetamine are: Risk of tolerance leading to dependence. Agitation, restlessness and insomnia. Headaches. Dizziness. Loss of appetite. Dry mouth. Diarrhoea or constipation. Difficulty with urination. In children, tearfulness, loss of appetite and loss of weight.

Conditions in which Dexamphetamine Must be Avoided

Heart disease. Glaucoma (a condition in which there is abnormally high pressure in the eye). Extrapyramidal disorders (disorders of those parts of the central nervous system which control certain muscular actions). Overexcited states. Thyrotoxis (a condition in which excessive amounts of thyroid hormones in the bloodstream cause rapid heart beat, tremors, anxiety, sweating, increased appetite, loss of weight and intolerance of heat). Where there is a history of drug dependency.

Conditions in which Dexamphetamine Should be Used with Caution

Insomnia. Caution is advised when used with antidepressants, anaesthetics, remedies for coughs and colds and treatments for high blood pressure.

PEMOLINE	
Trade name	*Description*
Volital	20 mg white tablets marked p9.

General Information

Pemoline is described as a weak CNS (central nervous system) stimulant and is suggested for the treatment of hyperactivity in children under specialist psychiatric supervision.

Dosage Information

Children: Over the age of six, between 6–10 mg, morning and afternoon.

Side Effects and Further Information

Pemoline has been described as having a stimulant effect somewhere between caffeine and amphetamines. It has a mild alerting effect and may give a feeling of well being. Side effects are said to be infrequent and mild, but it would be unwise and unhelpful for it to be taken too close to bedtime as it is likely to cause insomnia, its most common side effect. Other side effects which may be experienced are rapid heart beat, agitation and weight loss. Long-term use may retard growth in children.

Conditions in which Pemoline Must be Avoided

Glaucoma (a condition in which there is abnormally high pressure in the eye). Extrapyramidal disorders (disorders of those parts of the central nervous system which control certain muscular actions). Overexcited states. Thyrotoxis (a condition in which excessive amounts of thyroid hormones in the bloodstream cause rapid heart beat, tremors, anxiety, sweating, increased appetite, loss of weight and intolerance of heat).

Conditions in which Pemoline Should be Used with Caution

Insomnia. Caution is advised when used with antidepressants, anaesthetics, remedies for coughs and colds and treatments for high blood pressure.

PROLINTANE

Trade name	Description
Villescon	Red liquid containing prolintane and vitamins B and C.

General Information

The manufacturers recommend prolintane as a general 'pick-me-up' or tonic after 'illness, surgery, or labour, for apathy and anorexia in elderly patients, for institutional neuroses and for anorexia and lassitude following radiotherapy.' The British National Formulary specifically does not recommend prolintane. This preparation is a mild stimulant with the unusual effect for a drug in this group of stimulating rather than suppressing the appetite.

Dosage Information

10 ml twice daily before 4 pm.

Side Effects and Further Information

This drug is not available for prescription on the NHS. Its side effects of restlessness, agitation, excitability and upset stomach, are similar to other stimulants but much less severe and less frequent.

Getting the Most Out of Your Doctor

When you are prescribed a psychiatric drug it is important that you understand what the drug is, how you should take it and what effects it will have on you. You may wish to know whether there is any alternative treatment to the proposed drug. You may want to ask whether psychotherapy or some other form of psychological treatment is available, either as an alternative to the drug, or whether psychological help might help you to recover sooner. When you know all the facts you may decide against taking the drug and look for different ways of dealing with your problems. Depending on how serious your mental health problem is, it may be extremely unwise for you not to take the medication. Whenever any treatment is under consideration the balance of its benefits against its unwanted effects needs to be considered in making the decision. The following list of questions for your doctor should help you to make your decision and to get the most out of your treatment.

1. What and how?

*What kind of medicine is it?

*How can it help me?

*How and when should I take it?

*What should I do if I miss a dose?

*How will I know that it works?

2. How important is it?

*How important is it that I take it?

*What may happen if I do not take it?

3. What side effects?

*Does it have any side effects?

*How likely is it that I will experience these side effects?

*Does taking it for a long time have any risks or dangers?

*Can I drive whilst taking it?

*Can I drink alcohol whilst taking it?

*Is it safe to take other medicines whilst taking it?

*Are there any foods I should avoid whilst taking it?

4. How long?

*How long should I continue taking it?

*When will I need to see you again?

*What will you need to know when I see you again?

If you are worried about any aspect of the treatment or uncertain about the advice you have been given and are unable to resolve these with your doctor you may ask to be referred to another doctor for a second opinion.

Translating Your Prescription

When your doctor issues a prescription he may use the scholarly language of Latin to convey to the pharmacist instructions as to how and when the prescribed medication should be administered. The pharmacist then feeds these instructions into a computer which translates and prints them in modern English for you to read on a label. This quaint ritual is kept alive by a shrinking minority of doctors. The following glossary of the abbreviations used in prescriptions will help you to translate them, assuming of course, that you can read your doctor's handwriting!

a.c.	*ante cibos*	before meals
ad.	*ad.*	to make (a total)
ad. lib.	*ad libitum*	as much as required
b.d. **b.i.d.** **b.d.s.** }	*bis in die sumendum*	twice daily

c	*cum*	with
caps.	*capsules*	
c.m.s.	*cras mane sumendum*	take tomorrow morning
c.n.	*cras nocte*	take tomorrow evening
d. } **det.**	*detur*	give
e.m.p.	*ex modo prescripto*	as directed
f. **ft.**	*fiat*	make up
Gtt.	*guttae*	drops
g. or G,Gm	*grammum*	gram
haust.	*haustus*	draught
h.n.	*hac nocte*	tonight
hor. decub.	*hora decubitus*	at bedtime
h.s.	*hac nocte*	at bedtime
liq.	*liquor*	solution
m.et n.	*mane et nocte*	morning and evening
mane	*mane*	in the morning
m.d. } **m.d.u.**	*more docto utendum*	take as directed
mg. or mgm.	*milligrammum*	milligram(s)
mist.	*mistura*	mixture
ml.		millilitre(s)
mor. sol.	*more solito*	as usual
nocte	*nocte*	at bedtime
nocte. maneq.	*nocte maneque*	night and morning
n.r. } **non rep.**	*non repetatur*	do not repeat
o.m.	*omni mane*	each morning
o.n.	*omni nocte*	each night
p.c.	*post cibos*	after meals
p.p.a.	*phialla prius agitata*	shake the bottle
p.r.n.	*pro re nata*	when required
pulv.	*pulvis*	powder
q.h.	*quaque hora*	every hour
q.4.h.	*quaque 4 hora*	every 4 hours
q.d.	*quater in die*	

q.s.	quantum sufficiat	as much as required
rep.	repetatur	repeat
s.o.s.	si opus sit	when required
stat.	statim	at once
syr.	syrupus	syrup
tabs.	tabellae	tablets
t.d.	ter in die sumendem	three times daily
t.d.s.		
t.i.d.		
ung.	unguentum	ointment
ut dict.	ut dictum	as directed

Mental Health Treatment and the Law

Informed Consent in Psychiatric Treatment

In Britain the legal position on informed consent to treatment is not very clear. There is a legal requirement that consent to treatment should be based on the patient being informed as to the nature of the treatment, its purposes and any hazards associated with it. This does not mean, however, that the doctor must tell the patient about every conceivable risk attached to the treatment. He or she is only obliged to inform the patient of such risks in broad terms, and there is scope for the doctor to exercise professional judgement as to what the patient is told. A doctor may not obtain valid consent by deceiving a patient about the nature or effects of a treatment, and neither may he or she exercise force or duress to obtain such consent. In an emergency a particular treatment may be given if it is necessary to save a life. For example, a doctor may give treatment to an unconscious patient if in the doctor's judgement that treatment is necessary to save the patient's life, or to a seriously mentally ill person who is incapable of giving a valid consent.

The legal position of patients receiving treatment for a mental illness is more complicated than that of people being treated for other illnesses. A number of factors need to be taken into account. These are:

The severity of the symptoms: The symptoms of serious mental illness can be very distressing to the patient and those around him or her. The distress felt by the patient must be the first consideration, with that of relatives or other carers second. This is not to say that the distress of relatives or other carers is unimportant, rather, that those involved in giving treatment must be clear as to whose distress or anxieties are being dealt with. It is not acceptable to pressure a patient into taking a drug or a higher dose of a drug simply for the convenience of others. The distress experienced by the patient as a result of a drug's effects or side effects may far exceed any embarrassment or inconvenience caused to others.

The strain imposed on those who care for the patient: Serious mental illness can cause people to behave in disturbed, disruptive and occasionally dangerous ways. It may be necessary to protect families from intolerable strains imposed by such behaviour in order to protect that patient's place within the family.

The risk of leaving dangerous symptoms untreated: In some instances it is necessary to give treatment in order to safeguard the safety of the patient, as well as people.

The benefits of the treatment versus the disadvantages: As will be seen in this guide, the drugs used in psychiatry are not effective for all patients, and some of the drugs expose patients to risks without any realistic expectations of benefits being gained. For some patients the treatment may be worse than the illness, whilst for others the risks and side effects of the drugs may be a small price to pay for the relief they bring from tormenting or dangerous symptoms. The strategy of steadily increasing the doses of antipsychotic drugs when they have been shown to be ineffective is dangerous and unacceptable. There are situations in which physical restraint is more acceptable than attempts to stun people with powerful drugs.

Consent and the law

Only a very small proportion of people receiving treatment for mental illness are detained under the compulsory sections of the 1983 Mental Health Act. The minority who are liable to be detained may in certain circumstances be administered treatment without their consent. The position of patients subject to compulsory detention is set out later in this section.

All patients who are not subject to detention in hospital

under the provisions of the Mental Health Act can refuse any treatment which they would rather not have. They have the same rights as anyone else to give or withhold legally valid consent, and in theory they should give such consent before they are given any treatment. In practice, however, few are either asked for consent or informed of their rights. What usually happens is that their prescription or injection is given as a matter of routine. In hospitals the medication trolley is often wheeled into the ward and patients are expected to queue passively and accept their treatment. In psychiatry, if the law on consent to treatment was observed to the letter, considerable inconvenience would be caused to those who prescribe and administer treatments. If it was observed, however, it might in time do much to improve both the quality of treatment received and the quality of relationships between patients and staff, which might ultimately lead to patients complying with treatment more readily. The main components of informed consent are as follows:

Information: The patient must be given information on the nature and purpose of the treatment and any serious side effects or hazards (the doctor is not obliged to inform the patient of *every* possible side effect or hazard but must not deceive the patient. In the current state of law the doctor is allowed to exercise professional judgement as to how much information is actually given to the patient).

Competency: The patient must be able to understand the nature and purpose of the treatment. The fact that someone is suffering from a mental disorder does not automatically mean that he is incapable of understanding the issues involved, but obviously some people will be better able to understand than others. A young person over the age of 16 has the same rights in consent procedures as an adult. The position of young people below the age of 16 is unclear, but learned opinion is that under current law that children should be assumed to have the same rights as adults, unless it is clearly demonstrated that such a young person lacks the capacity to understand the issues involved. Factors which must be taken into account in these circumstances include the child's chronological age, his or her mental age and abilities, his or her mental condition and his or her capacity to make realistic and informed choices between the available alternatives.

Voluntariness: The patient must give consent without undue force, persuasion or influence being brought to bear. A consent obtained by fraud, deceit or threat is not legally valid and any person for administering treatment under such circumstances would be acting unlawfully.

The only circumstances in which a person not subject to detention under the Mental Act can be treated without a consent first being obtained are in circumstances of *urgent necessity*. For example, it would be lawful in an emergency to give a person suffering from mental illness in order to prevent that person from harming himself or other people. However such treatment can only be given for as long as it is necessary to bring the emergency to an end; the patient's consent must be obtained to continue treatment beyond that point.

Patients Subject to Detention Under the Provisions of the Mental Health Act 1983

People who are detained in hospitals under sections of the Mental Health Act for 72 hours or less, or remanded to hospital for a medical report, who are under guardianship or who are conditionally discharged from hospital, have the same right to refuse treatment as any other person. All other patients subject to detention in hospital may be given treatment without consent under the terms set out in Part IV of the Mental Health Act. Patients who are uncertain about their legal standing under the Act should seek clarification from the hospital staff.

Section 58 of the Mental Health Act is specifically concerned with drug treatments. Under this section patients subject to detention – with the exceptions mentioned above – can be given drugs *without* their consent for up to three months from the start of treatment. After three months, the treatment *cannot* continue unless: a) the patient gives a legally valid consent, or b) a doctor appointed by the Mental Health Act Commission (a special body set up to protect the rights of detained patients) certifies that the treatment is necessary.

Cases of Urgent Necessity

In cases of urgent necessity it is lawful to treat a mentally disordered person without that person's consent. In such cases the safeguards contained in Section 58 of the Mental Health Act and outlined do not apply. Section 62 of the Act sets out the terms of such urgent necessities as treatment which:

a) is immediately necessary to save the patient's life;

b) (not being irreversible) is immediately necessary to prevent a serious deterioration of his or her condition;

c) (not being irreversible or hazardous) is immediately necessary to alleviate serious suffering by the patient;

d) (not being irreversible or hazardous) is immediately necessary and represents the minimum interference necessary to prevent the patient from behaving violently or being a danger to himself or to others.

The terms 'irreversible and hazardous' are explained as follows:

Treatment is irreversible if it has unfavourable irreversible physical or psychological consequences and hazardous if it entails significant physical hazard.

The legal issues surrounding consent to treatment are extremely complex and patients or relatives who need advice can contact MIND's Legal and Welfare Rights Service at the address provided on p. 196.

Complaints Procedures

Tangled Channels: A Brief Outline of Treatment Complaints Procedures

As many people have found – at the cost of considerable frustration – the procedures for making a complaint about a doctor's clinical judgement are totally inadequate. It may take years of persistence to get a complaint heard or resolved and the odds are stacked against the complaining patient. Complaints about the clinical judgement of doctors are heard by other doctors and many people have found them to be extremely reluctant to criticise the work of their colleagues. In psychiatry the quality of prescribing practice is often very poor: pragmatism seems to prevail over good practice and professional collusion militates against change for the better. Added to this is the stigma which is attached to people who have been diagnosed as being mentally ill. Thus in 'confidential' meetings to which the complainant is not invited – terms such as 'paranoid', 'manipulative', 'obsessional', 'neurotic' and 'schizophrenic' are likely to punctuate the discussions of a grievance. Whatever meanings these terms may have in their strictly clinical context, they can also provide an easy way out to the negligent or bad psychiatrist. Negotiating the complex channels of complaints concerning the exercise of clinical judgement requires persistence, skill, planning, patience and a lot of good luck. Before describing these channels, a few trips on negotiating them might be helpful:

Make it simple: Complaints about medical treatment are seldom simple or straightforward and it is therefore essential to clarify and simplify them as much as possible. It may be that you feel badly treated by a number of people who were at some stage directly or indirectly involved in your treatment, but remember that it is easier, and more effective, to shoot one arrow at a time. To put your complaint about one psychiatrist within a diatribe against the state of British psychiatry as a whole, will not help you to get satisfaction.

Make it soon: The longer you leave it before you make your complaint the more difficult it will be to establish the facts. Institutions often have very short memories when things have gone wrong.

Get help: Get the help, advice and support of someone who is used to dealing with complaints procedures. Listen to his or her advice very carefully, and remember that although you have more knowledge of the people you are complaining about your adviser will probably know more about the people you are compaining to. Every procedure has its ground rules and traditions and your adviser will be able to help you negotiate these, and hopefully use them to your advantage.

Put it in writing and keep a copy: You need to be sure that your complaint does not get 'lost in the post', so put it in writing, date it and keep a copy. Keep copies of any correspondence or documents concerning your complaint in a file, and don't use that file as a beer mat – sometimes the appearance of a complaint may tilt the balance as to how the complaint is eventually dealt with.

Keep it brief: You may well feel moved to write a 50-page letter but it is unlikely that anyone will feel moved to read it. The longer your letter, the more likely you are to be written off as a 'nutcase'.

Don't overstate your case: Remember the value of understatement. The language you use in your complaint will create that vital first impression of what sort of person you are in the minds of those who are going to judge the merits of your complaint. Remember also that there are more cock-ups than conspiracies in life and more incompetents than conspirators in psychiatry.

Don't be bought off or bullied: If your complaint was serious, withdrawing it before it has been resolved may expose others to the same bad treatment of which you are complaining. *But*, it is sometimes graceful to accept a sincere apology.

Now, into the maze . . .

Clinical Judgement

Clinical judgement means a doctor exercising his or her professional judgement as to the most appropriate treatment or method of treatment for the individual in the circumstances which prevail at the time. In making such judgements doctors are guided by professional ethics, as set out in the Hippocratic Oath and other conventions, their knowledge of the patient's illness and circumstances, their training and knowledge of the treatments and services available to meet the patient's medical needs, the duties of care as set out in law, and respect for the patient's human dignity.

Making a Complaint About a Hospital Doctor's Clinical Judgement

In the first instance any complaint should be made to the consultant responsible for your treatment, to the District Health Authority (DHA), or to an officer of the DHA, such as the district general manager or administrator. If at this stage the complaint is not resolved to your satisfaction, you must renew your complaint in writing to any of the above who will then notify the Regional Medical Officer. He or she may or may not then refer it to two independent consultants from the same branch of medicine as that of the doctor against whom the complaint was made. These two independent doctors will review your complaint and reach an opinion which will then be conveyed to you. However, this procedure has no guarantee of independence and no non-medical scrutiny or review. Thus, if, for example, your complaint concerns drugs which were inappropriately prescribed for you in a 'megadose' or an 'irrational' combination, the chances are that in the 'clinical' opinion of the independent doctors your complaint will be judged to be unjustified. You will have reached the cul-de-sac at the end of a very short road.

Making a Complaint About Your Treatment in Hospital

If you wish to complain about a minor matter concerning your care in hospital you should take the matter up with the hospital, which has an obligation to listen sympathetically to your complaint and to try to resolve it. If at this point the complaint is not resolved to your satisfaction, you may then take it up directly with the Chair of the District Health Authority.

Complaining About Your General Practitioner

If you feel that your general practitioner has failed to provide you with the service that he or she should have done under the terms of his or her agreement with the Family Health Service Committee, you may ask that body to investigate your complaint. You must lodge your complaint in writing within eight weeks of the event you wish to complain about. The address of your local Family Health Service Committee can be found on the front of your NHS card, or you may get the address, as well as some advice and help in making the complaint, from your local Community Health Council. However, many people have found this procedure yet another short road which turns out to be a cul-de-sac.

The Family Health Service Committee does not deal with complaints about clinical judgement. If you have a complaint about the way your GP has exercised his or her clinical judgement, you may have to consider legal action or a complaint to the General Medical Council (see below).

Making a Complaint About the Professional Misconduct of a Doctor

Serious professional misconduct is not defined in law as it is a matter which may involve acts or omissions which are not in themselves unlawful. Thus, a doctor would be judged guilty of serious professional misconduct if he or she had a sexual relationship with a patient. Other examples of professional misconduct might be breaching a confidential relationship, carelessly or improperly prescribing drugs, and improperly issuing medical certificates. It may involve behaviour which is damaging to the reputation of the medical profession, such as indecency, dishonesty or personally abusing drugs. Complaints should be made to:

The General Medical Council,
44 Hallam Street, London W1N 6AE

Making a Complaint About the Professional Misconduct of a Registered or Enrolled Nurse

Complaints should be made to:

The English Board of Nursing, Midwifery and Health Visiting, Victory House, 170 Tottenham Court Road, London W1P 0HA

Making a Complaint About Compulsory Admittance to a Mental Hospital or any Treatment Received Whilst Detained in Hospital

In the first instance you must make any complaints about your detention or the treatment you received as a detained patient to the managers of the hospital in which you are **detained or subject to** detention. If you are not satisfied by the response from the hospital managers you can write directly to:

The Mental Health Act Commission,
Maid Marian House, 56 Houndsgate, Nottingham NG1 6BG

Complaints about medical treatment outnumber all the other 18 categories of complaints made to the Mental Health Act Commission. The Commission has no authority to investigate complaints made by the 90 per cent of mental hospital patients who are not subject to compulsory detention. These so-called 'informal' patients are treated as badly or as well as patients subject to detention, but they have no recourse to the Commission or any other similar body. Patients not subject to detention who wish to complain about their treatment in a mental hospital should refer to the other complaints procedures set out in this section.

Complaints About Maladministration in the National Health Service

In the first instance the complaint should be made to the General Manager of the Health Authority responsible for the service you wish to complain about. If you are dissatisfied with the response from the General Manager, or if he or she declines to investigate your complaint, you may write directly to:

The Health Service Commissioner for England,
Church House, Great Smith Street, London SW1P 3BW

Useful Books

On Depression

Dorothy Rowe: *The Way Out of Your Pain* (Routledge Kegan Paul). A well-written and readable book on depression and how to deal with it.

Kathy Nairn and Gerrilin Smith: *Dealing With Depression* (Women's Press Handbook Series). A lively and committed book which does not pull its feminist punches.

Dr Michael Bott and Derek Bowskill: *The Do-It-Yourself Mind Book* (Wildwood House). An interesting and informative book dealing with different mental health problems and their treatments.

Tony Lake; *Defeating Depression* (Penguin). A useful book which is good at describing depression.

On Schizophrenia

Richard Warner: *Recovery From Schizophrenia* (Routledge & Kegan Paul). A scholarly and exhaustive text which is immensely readable and useful as a source of information.

Carol L. M. Caton: *Management of Chronic Schizophrenia* (Oxford University Press). A thorough book which some readers may find hard going.

On Tranquillizers

Larry Neild: *Escape from Tranquillizers and Sleeping Pills* (Ebury Press). A practical and readable guide to getting off tranquillizers.

Shirley Tricket SRN: *Coming off Tranquillizers* (Thorsons). One of the first books on tranquillizer withdrawal which remains one of the best.

Valerie Curran and Sue Golombok: *Bottling It Up* (Faber and Faber). A good book which provides a withdrawal guide and information on tranquillizers and antidepressants.

Useful Addresses

MIND (The National Association for Mental Health), 22 Harley Street, London W1N 2ED.

Wales MIND, 23 St Mary Street, Cardiff CF1 2AA

Scottish Association for Mental Health, 40 Shandwell Place, Edinburgh, EH2 4RT.

National Schizophrenia Fellowship, 78/79 Victoria Road, Surbiton, Surrey.

The Manic Depression Fellowship, 13 Rosslyn Road, Twickenham, Middlesex TW1 ZAR.

The Northern Ireland Association for Mental Health, Beacon House, University Street, Belfast.

Index